Comparative Endocrinology of Animals

Edited by Edward Narayan

Published in London, United Kingdom

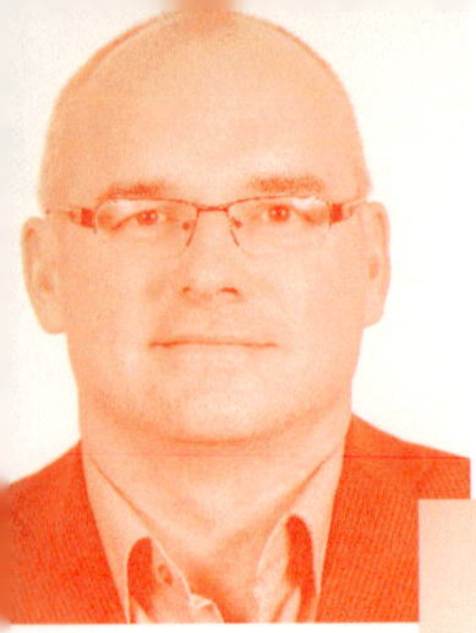
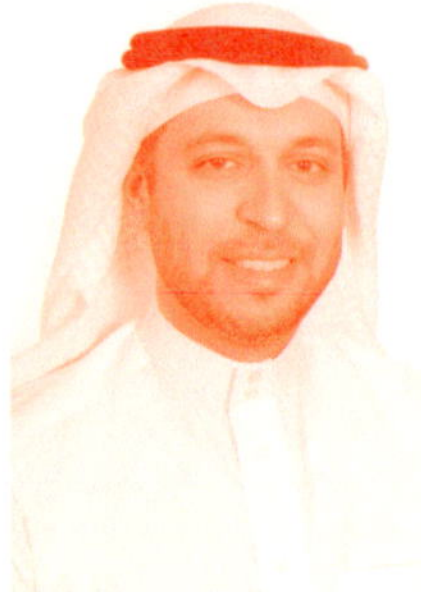
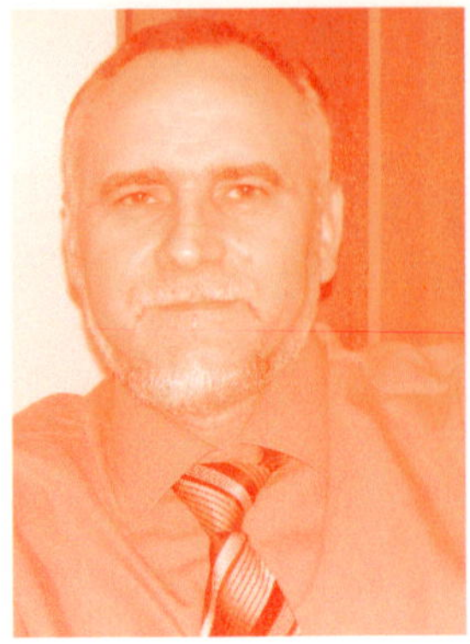
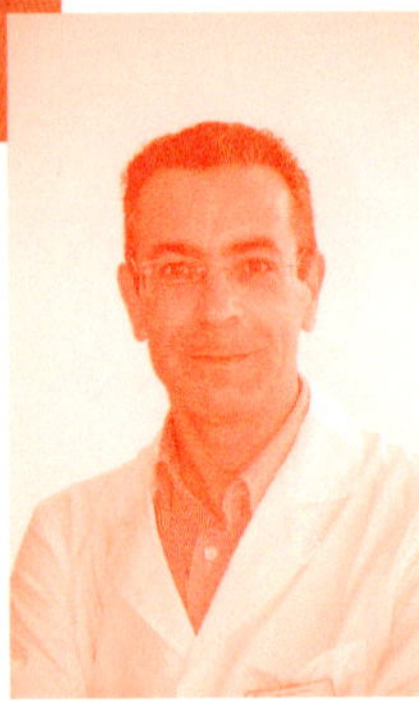
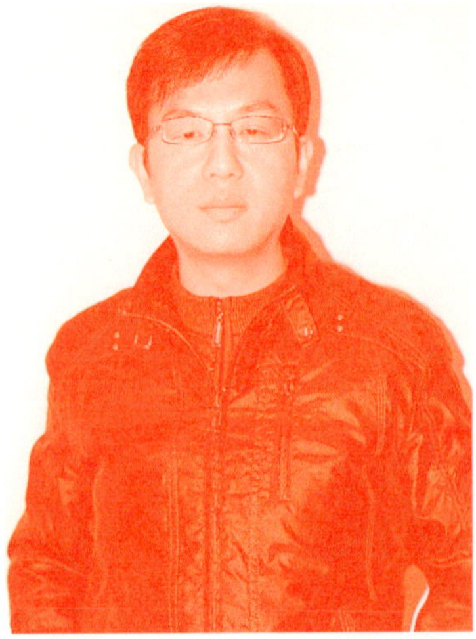
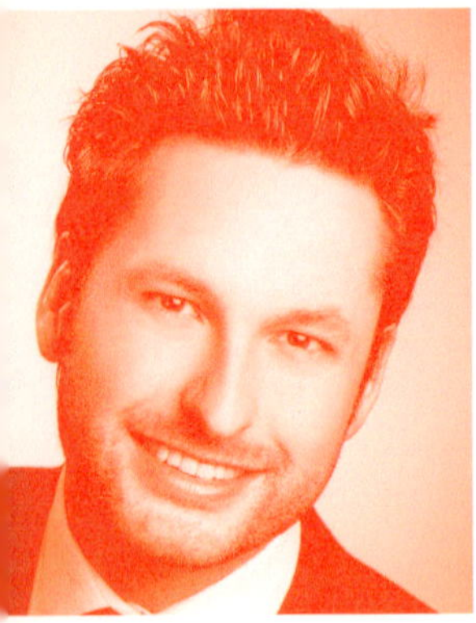
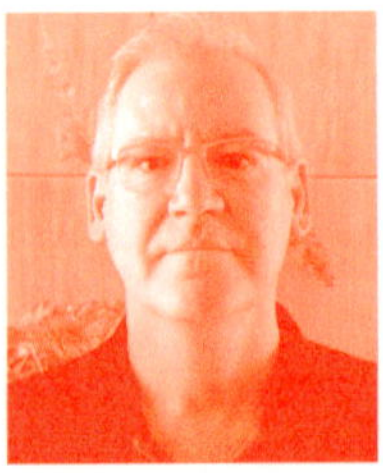

IntechOpen

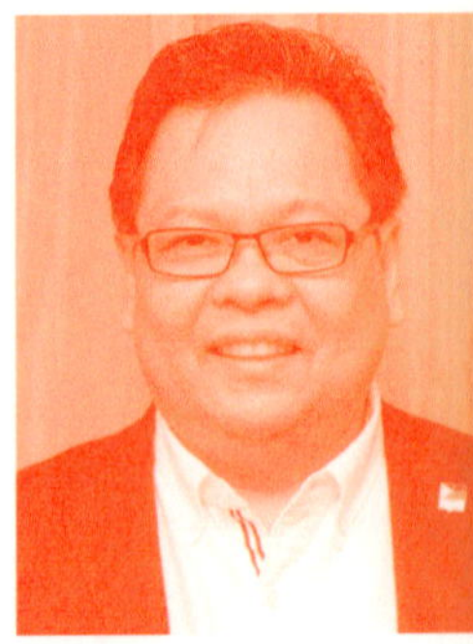
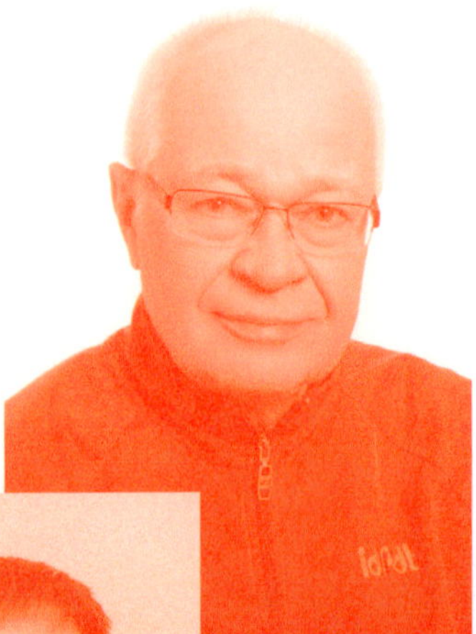
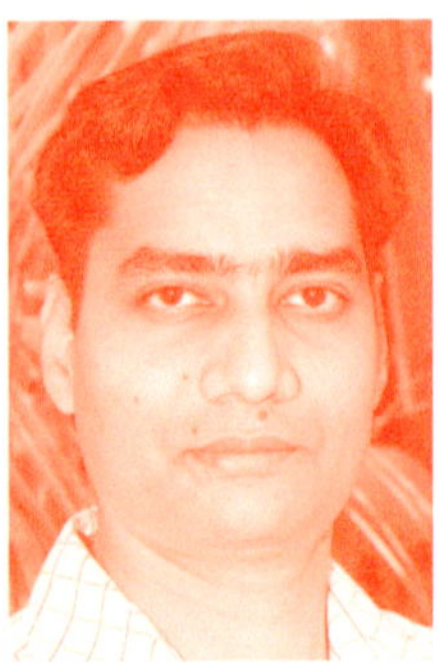
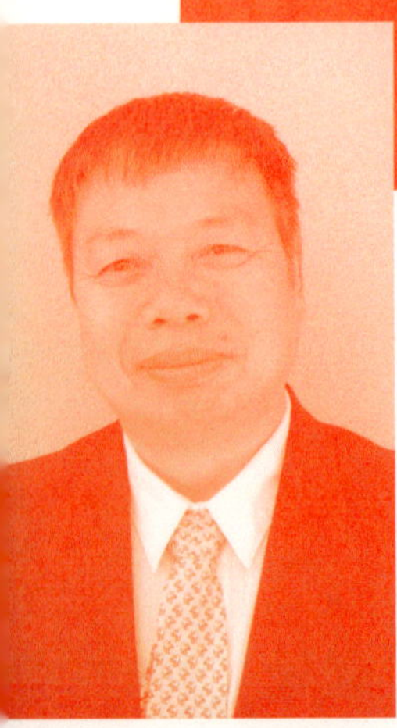
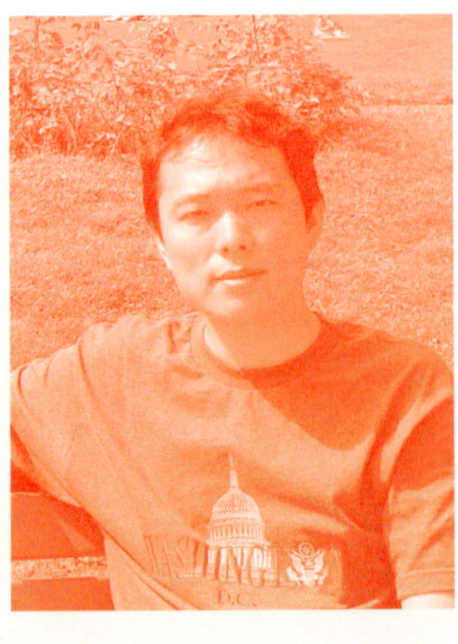
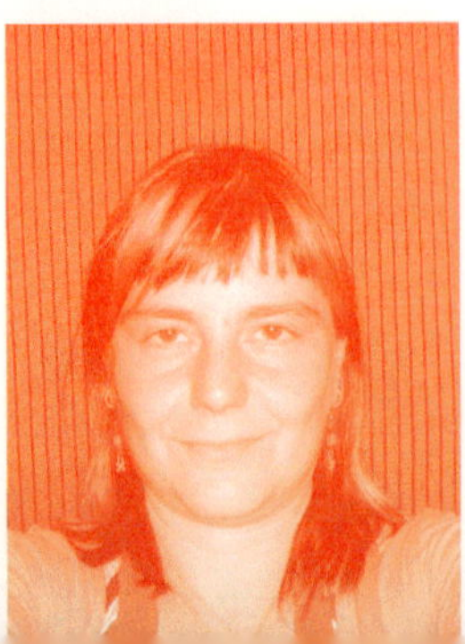

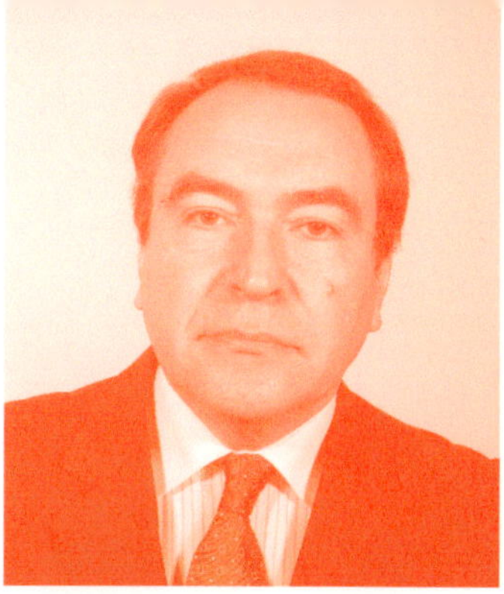
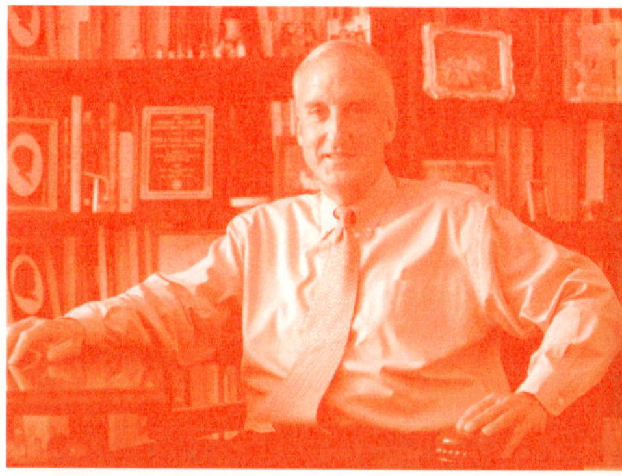
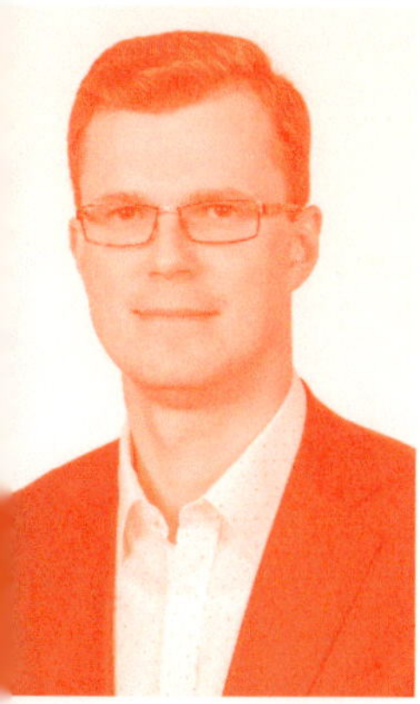
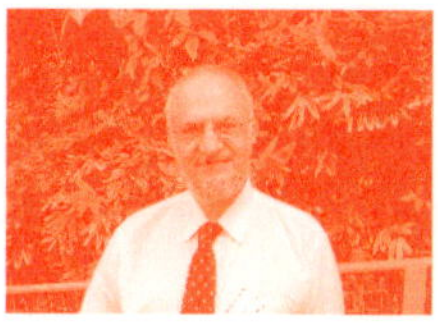
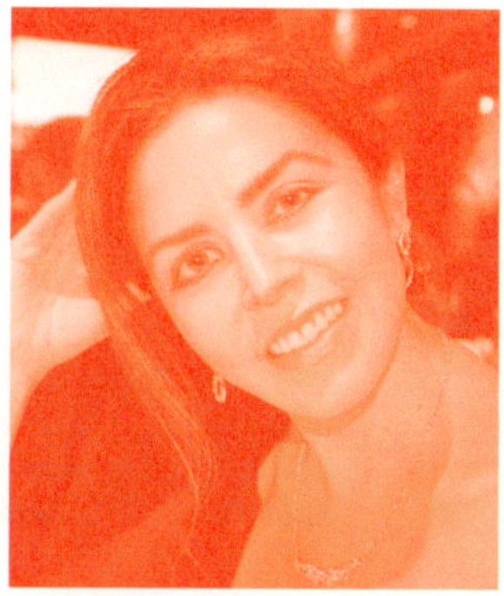

Supporting open minds since 2005

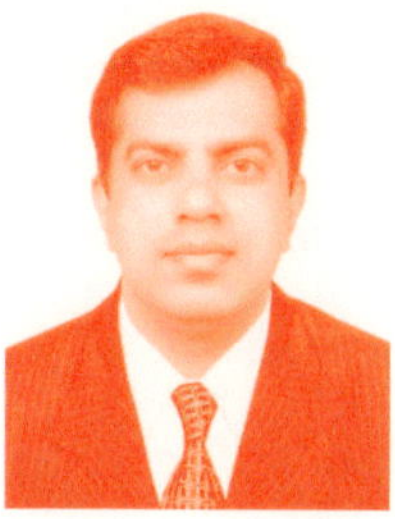
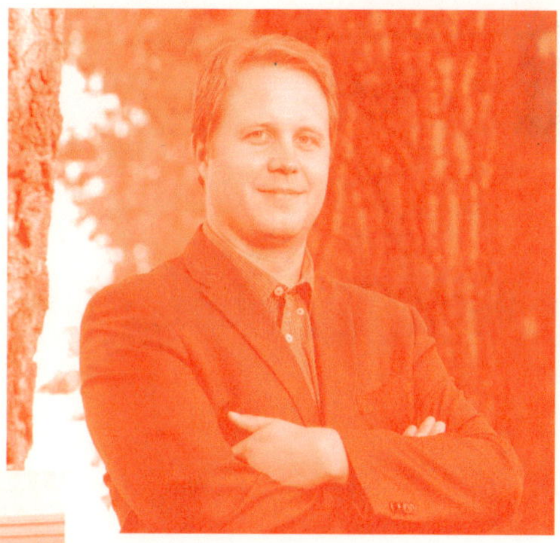
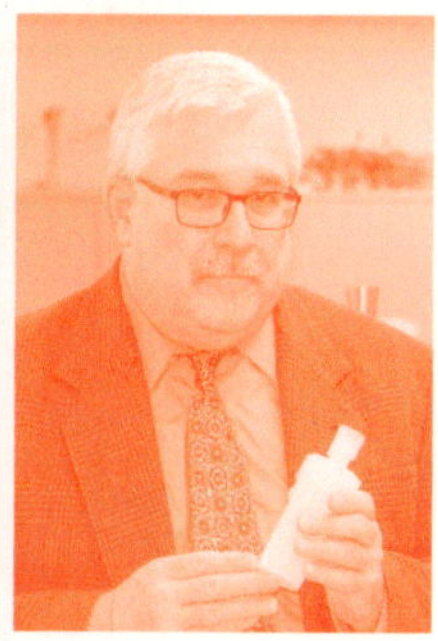
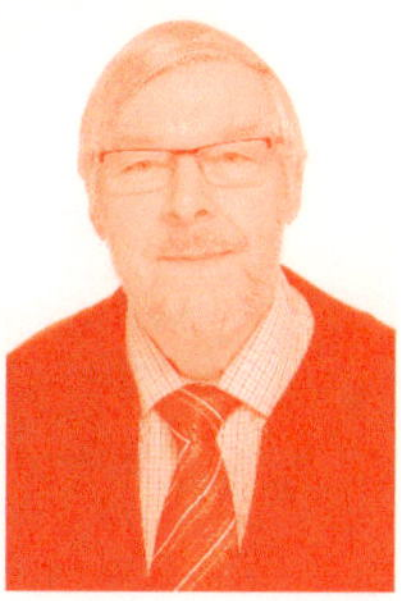
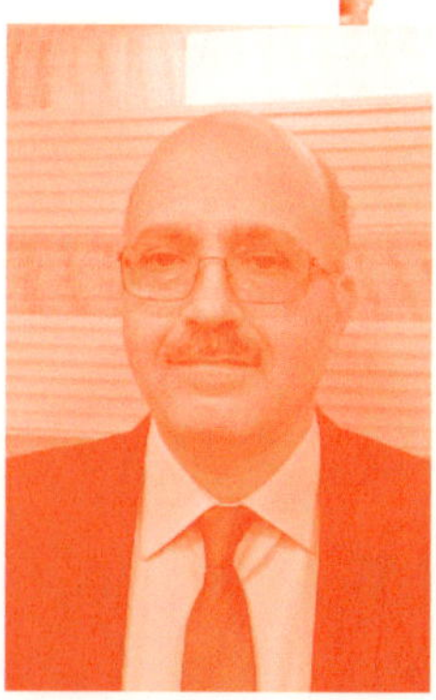
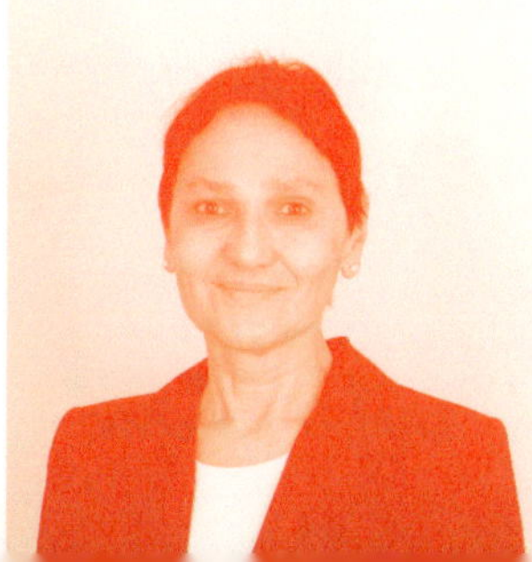
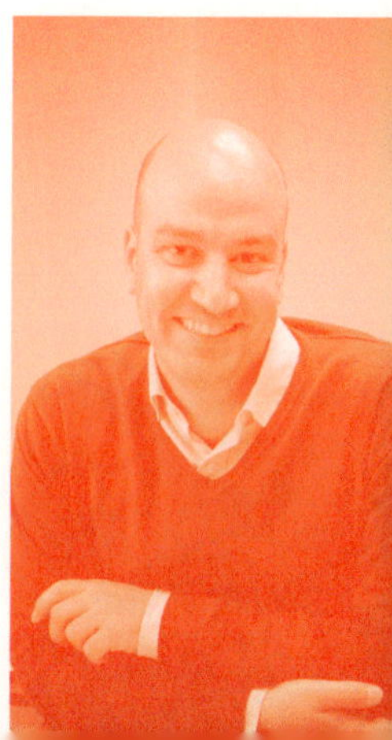

Comparative Endocrinology of Animals
http://dx.doi.org/10.5772/intechopen.73427
Edited by Edward Narayan

Contributors
Shui-Yuan Lu, Pinpin Lin, Chen-Yi Weng, Wei-Ren Tsai, Edward J Narayan, Gregory Sawyer, Ramachandra Reddy Pamuru, Alexandra Proshchina, Yuliya Krivova, Dmitriy Otlyga, Larisa Gurevich, Valeriy Barabanov, Iya Voronkova, Sergey Saveliev

First published in London, United Kingdom, 2019 by IntechOpen
IntechOpen is the global imprint of INTECHOPEN LIMITED, registered in England and Wales, registration number: 11086078, The Shard, 25th floor, 32 London Bridge Street
London, SE19SG – United Kingdom
Printed in Croatia

British Library Cataloguing-in-Publication Data
A catalogue record for this book is available from the British Library

Additional hard and PDF copies can be obtained from orders@intechopen.com

Comparative Endocrinology of Animals
Edited by Edward Narayan
p. cm.
Print ISBN 978-1-83880-396-4
Online ISBN 978-1-83881-194-5
eBook (PDF) ISBN 978-1-83881-195-2

For EU product safety concerns:
IN TECH d.o.o., Prolaz Marije Krucifikse Kozulić 3, 51000 Rijeka, Croatia, info@intechopen.com or visit our website at intechopen.com.

Meet the editor

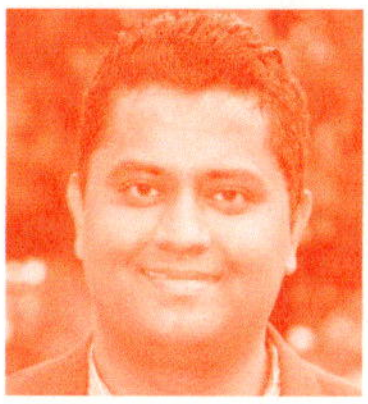

Editor Edward J. Narayan works as an animal biologist at the School of Science and Health of Western Sydney University. He earned his PhD in biology and has contributed to the establishment of noninvasive hormone monitoring technology to assess reproductive and stress hormones in amphibians. Dr. Narayan completed postdoctoral research in Australia and Canada and has had research stints in New Zealand and India. He has published over 70 peer-reviewed journal articles and supervised numerous masters and doctoral students in Australia and abroad. Dr. Narayan's current research program expands from wildlife conservation to production animals, and he directs the STRESS LAB at Western Sydney University.

Contents

Preface

Comparative endocrinology is an important component of animal physiology. Hormones influence animal physiology and behavior. Knowledge gained from studies in the hormonal biology of animals can be applied to the health management of diverse systems including production animals, wildlife species, and humans.

The contributing authors come from diverse science disciplines; herein they have applied comparative endocrinology approaches to the study of fundamental and applied areas such as aquaculture, livestock production, and human health management. The texts incorporated in the book are an attempt to provide a range of comparative endocrinology studies from crustaceans, rodents, ruminants, to humans. Each chapter author has provided robust datasets to support the research discussion and outcomes. The book will be useful to students of biological and biomedical sciences and to comparative physiologists, researchers, and clinicians.

The editor is thankful to every individual who helped in the preparation of this book, and he is indebted to the chapter contributors for accepting helpful criticism, resulting in the present shape of the book.

Last but not least, the editor thanks Ms. Manuela Gabric and Ms. Dajana Pemac, publishing process managers at IntechOpen, for sending information and guidelines that allowed this book's chapters to be edited well on time.

Dr. Edward Narayan
School of Science and Health, Western Sydney University,
New South Wales, Australia

Chapter 1

Introductory Chapter: Applications of Stress Endocrinology in Wildlife Conservation and Livestock Science

Edward Jitik Narayan

1. Introduction

Animals have contributed towards the progress of mankind in many ways such as through biomedicine, scientific research, domestication and farming, zoo animals and aquaculture [1–5]. The key concept of animal welfare underpins the quality of life of an animal while living under human management [6]. Animal welfare is a complex subject which takes into account the environmental and management factors that influence the physiological, behavioural and emotional (well-being or affective) state of animals [7, 8].

Animals such as elephants, dolphins, birds and dogs can display complex cognitive ability guided by processes such as perception, learning, memory and decision-making [9, 10]. Emotion in animals involves complex physiological, behavioural, immune, cognitive and morphological responses that enable them to generate behaviours to cope against stressors [11]. There are specific physiological markers of pain and stress that enable researchers to evaluate the welfare of animals from a quantitative viewpoint and relate the data to understand how the animal perceives its environment [12, 13].

2. Stress endocrine response

Disruption to an animal's homeostasis initiates activation of the hypothalamic-pituitary-adrenal (HPA) axis (**Figure 1**), the result of which generally prepares the body for some form of exertion [14, 15]. The hypothalamus releases corticotrophin-releasing hormone (CRH) [15], signalling the anterior pituitary to release adrenocorticotrophic hormone (ACTH) [15], which circulates in the blood resulting in an increased output of glucocorticoids from the adrenal cortex. Glucocorticoids, in which cortisol is pivotal to larger vertebrates and fishes, while corticosterone occurs mainly in birds, amphibians and reptiles, act to partition energy through gluconeogenesis, in preparation for a physical challenge, by diverting storage of glucose away from glycogen/fat and mobilising glucose from stored glycogen. Following the stress response, cortisol acts to initiate PH balance, as a blocker within a negative feedback process to CRH secretion, and motivates the animal to replenish energy stores and to restore homeostasis [16].

Under chronic stress, prolonged activation of the stress response will have deleterious downstream effects including the inhibition of normal reproductive function, suppression of the immune system, tissue atrophy and inhibition or abnormal growth rate (**Figure 1**). It can also lead to abnormal behaviours such as stereotypies [17].

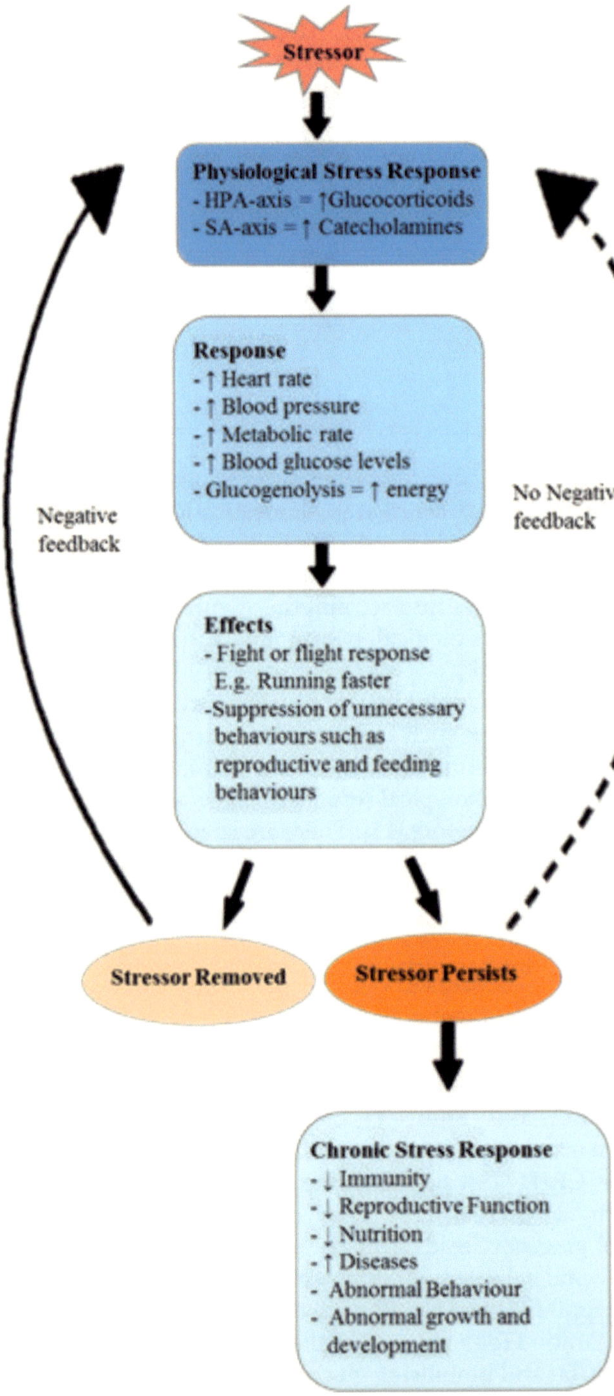

Figure 1.
Diagram demonstrating the generation of stress response under acute and chronic stress. Feedback loop for the HPA axis deactivation is shown using arrows.

3. Applications of stress hormone measurements

The present book has been focused on the applications of endocrine data in animal studies using examples from wildlife and production animals. Below I have provided examples of the stress hormone monitoring applied in wildlife and production animal research.

3.1 Wildlife translocation

Translocation programmes and captive breeding programmes are keys to species recovery [18]. Minimising the impact of multiple stressors on animals should be a major consideration when translocating animals from the wild into captivity and when maintaining animals in captivity [19]. Stress is a vital factor to consider when assessing animal welfare both in captivity and in the wild. Captive translocated animals are faced with a variety of stressors (i.e., factors that tend to change homeostasis) such as capture, transportation to release sites and captivity that may affect the settling of the animal into their new environment [20]. Short holding periods of animals can cause significant short-term stress responses, which may last for several days, weeks or months depending on the adaptive capacity of the species and the individual animals [21].

For example, the Fijian ground frogs (*Platymantis vitianus*) which IUCN listed as "endangered" species were translocated from their wild habitat into a captive breeding programme. As shown in **Figure 2**, the levels of stress hormone (corticosterone-indexed using urinary corticosterone metabolites) were elevated within 6 h post-translocation and remained elevated for up to 15 days before returning to pre-translocation levels.

3.2 Evaluation of stress in zoo wildlife

Animals in zoos encounter various environmental stimuli which may initiate a stress response such as noise, human interactions and climate [22, 23]. Stress hormone monitoring provides a quick and reliable quantitative way of assessing the stress responses of animals in zoos. An example is a study by the IUCN that listed marsupial,

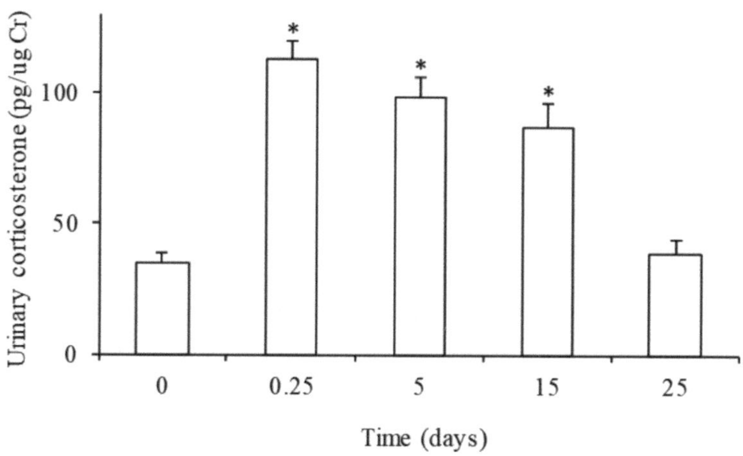

Figure 2.
Mean (+S.E.) urinary corticosterone in Fijian ground frogs. Sample sizes are N = 40 (for baseline urinary corticosterone), N = 10 per group for urinary corticosterone during transportation (6 h) and captivity at 5, 15 and 25 days.

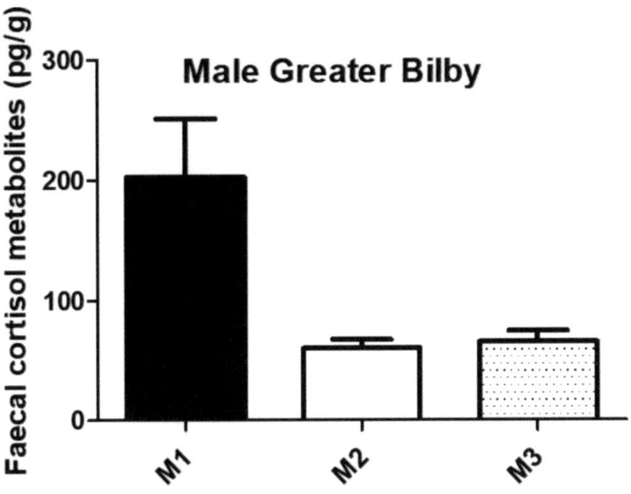

Figure 3.
Macrotis lagotis. Mean (±SEM) faecal cortisol metabolite profiles of male (N = 3) greater bilbies over the 21-day sampling period.

the greater bilby (*Macrotis lagotis*), as a "vulnerable" species. Using stress hormone monitoring through quantification of faecal glucocorticoid metabolites (FGMs) provided new knowledge on the stress responses of the bilbies to zoo activities and management interventions. As shown in **Figure 3**, the male bilbies showed variation in the levels of FGMs which was related to their health status and activity data.

Male 1 had chronic arthritis; however, males 2 and 3 showed no signs of illness or injury. Male 2 took part in activities such as shows, while male 3 did not. However, their mean FGM levels were apparently very similar (**Figure 3**).

3.3 Stress evaluation in farm animals

Stress can impact on the quality of livestock through effects on production traits such as growth and development, reproduction, meat quality, milk production and body condition [24–28]. Robust and sensitive non-invasive physiological tests that can detect subtle changes in the HPA axis activity to acute physical or psychological stressors in livestock are the focus of our research programme. Currently animals with the red meat, dark cutters are not identified until carcase assessment post-slaughter. The industry is seeking a preslaughter method to identify animals that are likely to produce dark meat (DC), which could allow either preslaughter intervention such as drafting out and preventative treatment of individuals or post-slaughter intervention.

A number of possible technologies exist, such as non-invasive faecal cortisol monitoring. Cortisol testing is considered paramount to the behavioural stress response because studies have found a good degree of positive association between traditional measurements of fear behaviour, body temperature and blood cortisol profiles in cattle [29]. Furthermore, individual differences in stress responses at slaughter may explain differences in rate or extent of pH decline between animals from a similar genetic and rearing background, slaughtered under similar conditions.

Dark-cutting or non-compliant beef is defined from the loin muscle (longissimus thoracis) having an ultimate pH (pHu) >5.7 or an AUSMEAT colour score >3 (Meat Standards Australia (MSA)). The major determinant of pHu is the concentration of muscle glycogen (muscle sugar) at slaughter. In the muscle post-mortem, glycogen forms lactic acid, which is correlated with the pH decline that occurs at

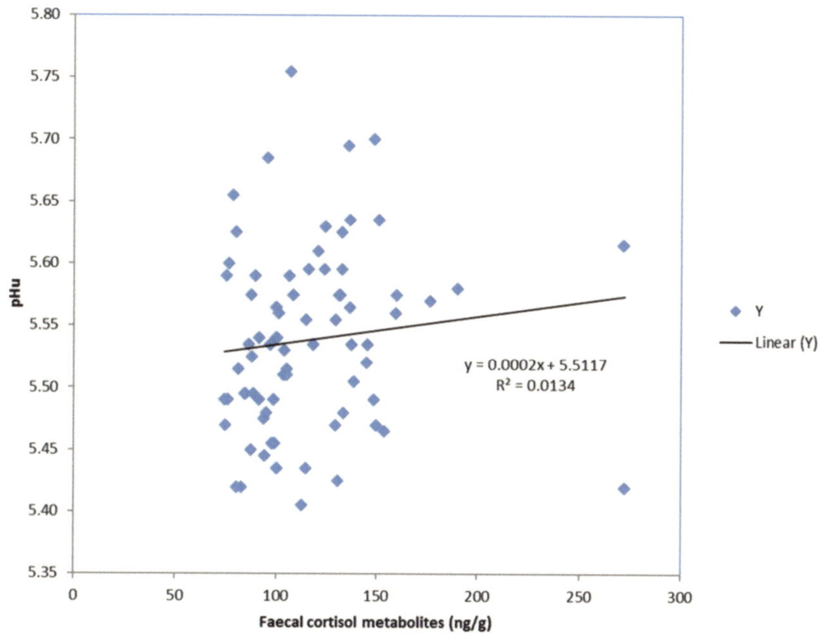

Figure 4.
Correlation between stress and ultimate pH of red meat using example of second-cross lambs. Both traits measured post-slaughter.

post-mortem. Lactic acid is one of the major contributors of lowered pH of the muscle from a pH of around 7, which is standard in a living animal, down to a pHu of around 5.4–5.7 within 24 h. If there is an insufficient muscle glycogen concentration at slaughter, there is limited formation of lactic acid, resulting in a high pHu and dark meat. Consumers do not like the appearance of dark beef, and high pH meat has shorter shelf-life and is unsuitable for vacuum packaging due to high susceptibility of spoilage [30].

Research with second-cross lambs demonstrated strong correlation between post-slaughter faecal cortisol metabolites and lamb meat quality traits, such as pHu—an indicator of dark-cutting (**Figure 4**). This positive correlation indicates that input of more stress on the farm could reduce meat quality through increased pH of red meat.

4. Conclusion

The above case studies demonstrate the wider applications of stress endocrinology in wildlife and production animal science. Hormone monitoring provides a useful tool for evaluating the health and welfare of animals when used in combination with health, behaviour and other relevant husbandry information.

Acknowledgements

The author is thankful to the university and industry collaborations; postgraduate students in Griffith University, Charles Sturt University, Western Sydney University, Massey University, Queensland University, NSW Department of Primary Industries and Dreamworld Themepark; and members of the Zoo and Aquarium Association (Australia).

Author details

Edward Jitik Narayan
School of Science and Health, Western Sydney University, Penrith, NSW, Australia

*Address all correspondence to: e.narayan@westernsydney.edu.au

References

[1] Robinson HJ. Animal experimentation leading to the development of drugs benefiting human beings and animals. American Journal of Public Health and the Nations Health. 1967;**57**(9):1613-1620

[2] Durning AB, Brough HB. Taking Stock: Animal Farming and the Environment. Washington, D.C., USA: Worldwatch Institute; 1991

[3] Hanson E. Animal Attractions: Nature on Display in American Zoos. Princeton, New Jersey, United States: Princeton University Press; 2004

[4] Tidwell JH, Allan GL. Fish as food: Aquaculture's contribution: Ecological and economic impacts and contributions of fish farming and capture fisheries. EMBO Reports. 2001;**2**(11):958-963

[5] Festing MFW, Butler W. International Index of Laboratory Animals: Giving Sources and Locations of Animals used in Laboratories Throughout the World. 3 ed. Carshalton, Surrey: Laboratory Animals Centre; 1975

[6] Green TC, Mellor DJ. Extending ideas about animal welfare assessment to include 'quality of life' and related concepts. New Zealand Veterinary Journal. 2011;**59**(6):263-271

[7] Broom DM. Animal welfare: Concepts and measurement. Journal of Animal Science. 1991;**69**(10):4167-4175

[8] Moberg GP, editor. Animal Stress. Switzerland AG: Springer; 2013

[9] Shettleworth SJ. Animal cognition and animal behaviour. Animal Behaviour. 2001;**61**(2):277-286

[10] Alerstam T et al. Migration along orthodromic sun compass routes by Arctic birds. Science. 2001;**291**:300-303

[11] Colditz IG, Hine BC. Resilience in farm animals: Biology, management, breeding and implications for animal welfare. Animal Production Science. 2016;**56**(12):1961-1983

[12] Mouraux A, Iannetti GD. The search for pain biomarkers in the human brain. Brain. 2018;**141**(12):3290-3307

[13] Huggett RJ. Biomarkers: Biochemical, Physiological, and Histological Markers of Anthropogenic Stress. United States: CRC Press; 2018

[14] Hing S, Narayan E, Thompson A, Godfrey S. A review of factors influencing the stress response in Australian marsupials. Conservation Physiology. 2014;**2**(1):1-17

[15] Whirledge S, Cidlowski JA. Glucocorticoids, stress, and fertility. Minerva Endocrinologica. 2010;**35**(2):109

[16] Romero MF. In the beginning, there was the cell: Cellular homeostasis. Advances in Physiology Education. 2004;**28**(4):135-138

[17] Meehan CL, Garner JP, Mench JA. Environmental enrichment and development of cage stereotypy in Orange-winged Amazon parrots (*Amazona amazonica*). Developmental Psychobiology. 2004;**44**(4):209-218

[18] Fischer J, Lindenmayer DB. An assessment of the published results of animal relocations. Biological Conservation. 2000;**96**(1):1-11

[19] Narayan E, Hero JM. Urinary corticosterone responses and haematological stress indicators in the endangered Fijian ground frog (*Platymantis vitiana*) during transportation and captivity. Australian Journal of Zoology. 2011;**59**(2):79-85

[20] Teixeira CP, De Azevedo CS, Mendl M, Cipreste CF, Young RJ. Revisiting translocation and reintroduction programmes: The importance of considering stress. Animal Behaviour. 2007;**73**(1):1-13

[21] Franceschini MD, Rubenstein DI, Low B, Romero LM. Fecal glucocorticoid metabolite analysis as an indicator of stress during translocation and acclimation in an endangered large mammal, the Grevy's zebra. Animal Conservation. 2008;**11**(4):263-269

[22] Morgan KN, Tromborg CT. Sources of stress in captivity. Applied Animal Behaviour Science. 2007;**102**(3-4):262-302

[23] Mason GJ. Species differences in responses to captivity: Stress, welfare and the comparative method. Trends in Ecology & Evolution. 2010;**25**(12):713-721

[24] Von Borell E. Neuroendocrine integration of stress and significance of stress for the performance of farm animals. Applied Animal Behaviour Science. 1995;**44**(2-4):219-227

[25] Das R, Sailo L, Verma N, Bharti P, Saikia J. Impact of heat stress on health and performance of dairy animals: A review. Veterinary World. 2016;**9**(3):260

[26] West JW. Effects of heat-stress on production in dairy cattle. Journal of Dairy Science. 2003;**86**(6):2131-2144

[27] Maurya VP, Sejian V, Kumar D, Naqvi SMK. Impact of heat stress, nutritional restriction and combined stresses (heat and nutritional) on growth and reproductive performance of Malpura rams under semi-arid tropical environment. Journal of Animal Physiology and Animal Nutrition. 2016;**100**(5):938-946

[28] Ferguson DM, Warner RD. Have we underestimated the impact of pre-slaughter stress on meat quality in ruminants? Meat Science. 2008;**80**(1):12-19

[29] Voisinet BD, Grandin T, O'Conner SF, Tatum JD, Deesing MJ. *Bos indicus*-cross feedlot cattle with excitable temperaments have tougher meat and a higher incidence of borderline dark cutters. Meat Science. 1997;**46**(4):367-377

[30] ANON. Meat Research Newsletter. CSIRO Division of Food Research No. 84/l; 1984

Chapter 2

Ontogeny of the Human Pancreas

Alexandra E. Proshchina, Yuliya S. Krivova, Larisa E. Gurevich, Valeriy M. Barabanov, Dmitriy A. Otlyga, Iya A. Voronkova and Sergey V. Saveliev

Abstract

Pancreatic disorders are the most common pathologies in humans worldwide. Detailed information on pancreatic cytoarchitecture, vascularisation, innervation, morphogenesis, and cell differentiation is required for the development of new approaches to the treatment of these diseases. Currently, the majority of studies on pancreas development are performed on experimental animals (mainly rodents). Studies on human pancreatic prenatal development are restricted in number by ethical constraints and some technical difficulties. However, interspecies differences in pancreatic structure and development are considerable. Therefore, data obtained in experiments on animals and cell cultures must be supplemented with information obtained directly from human pancreatic autopsies. In this chapter, we summarise our previous results and the literature data on human pancreatic ontogeny. Special attention has been paid to the endocrine pancreas, which undergoes morphogenetic restructuring during human development. Several forms of structural organisation of the endocrine pancreas (single endocrine cells, small clusters of endocrine cells, mantle, bipolar, and mosaic islets) gradually appear during development. It is important that this restructuring is accompanied by changes in the ratio of pancreatic endocrine cells. The mechanisms of these changes are still unclear. The difficulties in identifying progenitor cells and tracking cell differentiation are the main problems associated with this issue.

Keywords: pancreas, islets of Langerhans, human development, transcription factors, Nkx6.1, Neurod1

1. Introduction

The pancreas is a unique organ that combines both endocrine and exocrine functions, which determines the diversity of its pathology. Pancreatic disorders (such as malignant neoplasms, pancreatitis, and diabetes mellitus) are the most common pathologies in humans worldwide. For example, according to the International Diabetes Federation, worldwide, 10% of adults will have type 1 or 2 diabetes by 2030 [1]. Currently, there are not enough effective methods of diabetes treatment aimed at replenishing and maintaining the population of insulin-producing cells. New techniques for the recovery of islet cells based on the natural mechanisms of the endocrine cell pool renewal are required.

For a long time, it was believed that the ability of the pancreas to respond to insulin demands is very limited during life. Recently, evidence of pancreatic endocrine part plasticity has been found, indicating that the number of β-cells varies under the influence of some physiological parameters. For example, it increases in cases of altered metabolic demand such as pregnancy and obesity, as well as during normal physiological growth [2, 3]. According to the literature, mechanisms of pancreatic β-cell plasticity are associated with the processes of cell proliferation, cell death, neogenesis, and changes in cell volume [4–6]. Recent work in rodents has indicated a previously unappreciated proliferative capacity of β-cells. However, the age of the animal appears to play a central role in determining the proliferative capacity of β-cells, as older animals display a significant decline in cellular expansion [7]. At the same time, the endocrine pancreas consists not only of β-cells but also contains several types of endocrinocytes. The endocrine cells of the pancreas are grouped into formations called pancreatic islets, but the details of the mechanisms and stages of human islet morphogenesis are still not fully resolved [8, 9].

All basic cell types of the pancreas originate from a single pluripotent cell with ductal phenotype [10–14]. It has been suggested that, in addition to the proliferation of existing β-cells, new cells can be obtained from differentiated adult pancreatic cells by interconverting between endocrine and exocrine parts. There are also suggestions regarding ontogenesis from duct cells or from other progenitor cells [6, 15]. Acinar cells are another potential source of new pancreatic endocrine cells. So-called acino-insular cells have been identified in many vertebrate species [16]. These cells simultaneously contain granules with digestive enzymes and granules containing hormones.

Recently, along with hypotheses about the replication of β-cells and the neogenesis of islets from progenitor stem cells, the hypothesis of transdifferentiation of some insulin-containing cells into glucagon-containing cells and the reverse transformation have been suggested [17, 18]. Most of these studies have been conducted on rodents, and there is still not enough data to confirm the existence of such mechanism in humans. However, in the endocrine cells of the developing human pancreas, co-expression of several hormones has been observed (see below). Some researchers believe that, in the human pancreas, these cells may be the precursors of endocrine cells [8].

It is also necessary to emphasise the importance of research directly on human pancreas samples. Currently, most studies into pancreas development are performed on experimental animals (mainly rodents) and cell cultures. However, adult β-cells have a limited lifespan in culture and undergo dedifferentiation, with the loss of insulin expression [7]. Interspecies differences in pancreatic structure and development are also considerable. For example, the formation of pancreatic islets in rodents is observed only in the first 2 weeks after birth, whereas, in the developing human pancreas, islets can be observed starting from 12 weeks of gestational development. Differences in the structure of the endocrine part of the pancreas in rodents and humans are also considered. In rodents, islets have a mantle-type structure, in which glucagon (α)- and somatostatin (δ)-containing cells are located at the islet periphery, and β-cells occupy the central part of the islet. In humans, islets of a mixed type are characteristic, in which α- and δ-cells can be not only at the periphery but also in the centre of the islet. In addition, bipolar islets (β-cells located at one pole of the islet and α- and δ-cells at another) are present during prenatal human development. In rodents, this stage of islet development has not been identified. Therefore, data obtained in experiments on animals and cell cultures must be supplemented with information obtained directly from the human pancreas. Although the basic developmental programme may be similar, the identity and/or timing of activity of some factors may be critically different.

In this chapter, we summarise our previous results and the literature data on the ontogeny of the human pancreas. We examined pancreatic autopsies derived from human foetuses from the 10th to the 40th week of development and from adults, using histological, IHC, and morphometric methods.

2. Pancreas structure in adults

The human pancreas is a well-defined unpaired elongated organ, in which three parts are usually distinguished: the head, body, and tail.

The pancreas combines both endocrine and exocrine functions. The exocrine compartments are identified as acinar and ductal cells. Acinar cells synthesise digestive enzymes that aid in nutrient metabolism, and ductal cells line the channels that transport these secretions to the gastrointestinal tract. The human exocrine pancreas (together with the mesenchyme) occupies 96–99% of the total pancreas volume [19, 20]. The endocrine pancreas occupies 1–4% of the total human pancreas volume. The main function of the endocrine pancreas is the regulation of carbohydrate metabolism. The mammalian (and human) endocrine pancreas contains four main types of endocrine cells: β-cells that produce, store, and secrete insulin (51 amino acid residues); α-cells that produce, store, and secrete glucagon (29 amino acid residues); δ-cells that produce, store, and secrete somatostatin (14 amino acid residues); and PP-cells that produce, store, and secrete pancreatic polypeptide (36 amino acid residues). The fifth type of pancreatic endocrine cells is the ghrelin-containing cells (ε), which are present in small numbers in the developing pancreas but disappear after birth [21, 22]. In the endocrine pancreas of some mammals, two other cell types have been described: EC-cells, which synthesise serotonin, and G-cells, which contain gastrin. These cells are extremely rare and can be found only at some stages of prenatal development.

However, this scheme is probably oversimplified. Recent studies have spurred an intense debate about whether β-cells represent a single homogeneous population or consist of subpopulations with functional and molecular variations to facilitate specialised tasks and responses to changes in the physiological environment [23].

In addition, several basic forms of endocrine pancreas structural organisation have been identified in the human pancreas (**Figure 1**): single endocrine cells, small clusters of cells, small islets of the mantle type, and large mosaic (mixed) islets [24–26]. The adult human pancreas contains from 100,000 to 2,000,000 islets [27], each of which contains from several hundreds to several thousands of endocrine cells. Large islets have a developed capillary network and are surrounded by a capsule. In humans, mice, and some other studied animals, the maximum islet size is about 500 microns [28, 29]. In addition, as mentioned above, acino-insular single cells have been identified in the pancreas of many vertebrates [16].

In mantle-type islets (**Figure 1c**), β-cells predominate and occupy the central islet part, while other cell types (α-, δ- and PP-cells) are located on the islet periphery. In our previous study, it was shown that the diameter of such islets in humans is less than 100 microns. In rodents (e.g. mice and rats), pancreatic islets of the mantle type are characteristic [30, 31], and mosaic islets (**Figure 1d**) are characteristic in the human pancreas [25, 31, 32]. However, in our study, it was shown that, in adults not suffering from disorders of carbohydrate metabolism, the contribution of the mantle type islets to the islet number was up to 65% of all insulin-containing cells. Islets with diameter more than 100 microns (i.e. mixed islets, since bipolar islets have not been identified in adults) represent only 10–15% of all islets, although they contain up to 35–40% of all the β-cells in the human endocrine pancreas. Similar data were obtained by Kilimnik et al. [26]. Moreover, it is believed that, in mosaic

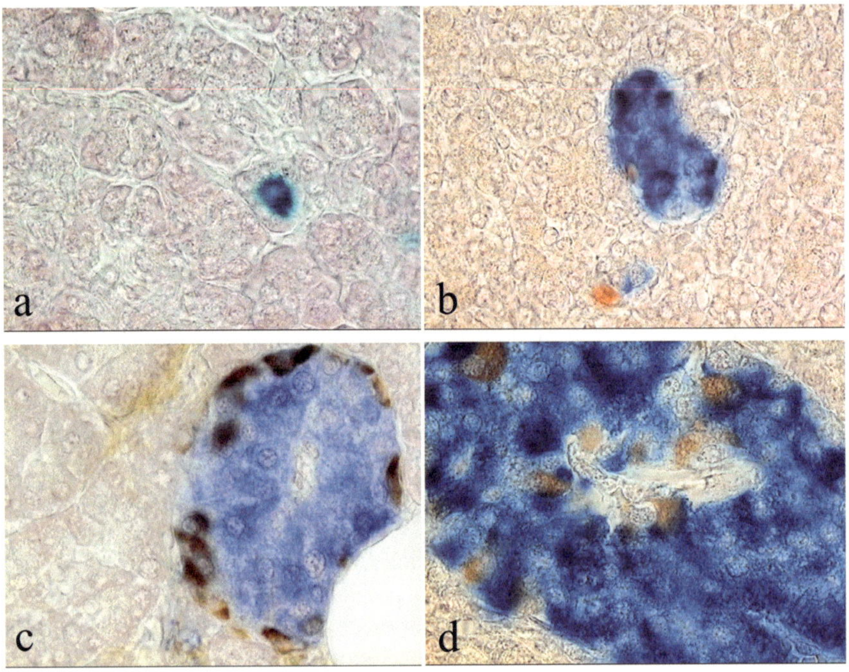

Figure 1.
Forms of endocrine pancreas structural organisation in adults (women, 75 years of age): (a) single endocrine cell, (b) small cluster of endocrine cells, (c) islet of mantle type, and (d) fragment of mosaic islet. Double immunohistochemical labelling with antibodies to glucagon (red) and insulin (blue), objective x100.

islets, the cells are located without clear ordering. In some studies [25, 33, 34], it was indicated that mixed (mosaic) islets of Langerhans have a clear, ordered structure. Within these islets, segments restricted by blood vessels have been identified. β-cells are located in the central part of the lobules, while α- and δ-cells are located at the periphery and around blood capillaries.

In humans, the main mechanism by which the endocrine pancreas grows during the neonatal period is an increase in the islet size rather than their number [35, 36], i.e. a 10% increase in the β-cell mass occurs in a small proportion (10%) due to the formation of new islets and to a much greater proportion (90%) due to an increase in islet size. It is important to note that, during adolescence in humans, no significant changes in islet number or cellular architecture have been detected.

The endocrine pancreas is also affected by the exocrine pancreas, as well as the vascular, lymphatic, and nervous systems. For example, according to some authors, nervous system structures are the first target of an autoimmune attack in type 1 diabetes [37]. At the same time, relatively little is known about these interactions, especially in humans [38].

Thus, information on the cellular composition of pancreatic islets in humans and the contribution of different types of hormone-secreting cells to the plasticity of the endocrine pancreas is contradictory. The main focus of studies devoted to this issue has been on insulin-secreting cells. However, the intimate arrangement of heterogeneous cells in islets has been implicated in the functional regulation of islets [39]. The mechanisms responsible for changes in the number and ratio of endocrine cells are still unclear [4–6]. Therefore, it seems logical to examine these issues during prenatal human development.

3. Prenatal development of the human pancreas

All parenchymal cell types of the pancreas (acinar, ductal, and endocrine cells) are derived from primitive endodermal cells of the foregut. After gastrulation, the thickened endodermal epithelium along the dorsal and ventral surfaces of the posterior foregut gives rise to the pancreas. In humans, the pancreas originates from the two primary diverticula of the primitive gut at 26 days postconception (d.p.c.; ≈6 weeks of gestational development) [40]. The epithelia of the gut evaginate into the surrounding mesoderm-derived mesenchymal tissue and form dorsal and ventral pancreatic buds. In some studies, two ventral buds are described. However, the left ventral bud gradually regresses, whereas the right ventral bud starts to migrate posteriorly. According to several reports, failure of the left ventral bud to regress could lead to the pathological condition known as annular pancreas (reviewed in [41]).

These buds continue to expand, branch, and fuse as a result of the gut rotation that brings the buds together [7]. The parenchyma of the two buds merges during the 7th week of gestation. The ventral pancreas gives rise to the ventral or lower part of the head of the pancreas, whereas the dorsal pancreas gives rise to the dorsal or upper part of the head, the body, and the tail. Together with the parenchyma, the ducts of the primitive pancreas also merge (for more details, see [42]). Many factors are involved in these processes, including interactions with the mesenchyme and expression of pancreas-specific transcription factors (see below) [43].

The branching of the human pancreatic epithelium to form the duct system starts at the end of the embryonic period (56 d.p.c.) [8, 40, 44]. At 7 weeks of gestation, a network of tubes of undifferentiated epithelial cells forms, from which the endocrine and exocrine components of the pancreas derive. Thus, in the prenatal period, both endocrine and exocrine cells originate from cells located in the primitive pancreatic ducts.

The endocrine pancreas starts to develop earlier than the exocrine acini. Typical pancreatic lobes form only at 14–16 weeks of gestation. This process becomes more accentuated and dense at the tissue periphery and then throughout the gland between gestational week 25 and gestational week 41 [41].

Data on the timing of appearance of the major types of hormone-containing cells are contradictory; some authors suggest that the glucagon- [45, 46] or somatostatin-containing cells [47] are detected first during human pancreas morphogenesis. However, most authors have identified β-cells first. So, in the studies of Polak et al. [48] and Piper et al. [40], hormone expression, evident as rare epithelial cells immunoreactive for insulin, was first apparent at 10 weeks of gestational development (at 52 d.p.c). One week later (immediately after the embryonic period) at 8.5 weeks postconception (w.p.c.; ≈ 11 weeks of gestational development), glucagon and somatostatin were detected separately in isolated pancreatic epithelial cells. PP-containing cells were identified only at 12 weeks. Data obtained in a study by Jeon et al. [8] are similar: the first insulin-positive cells were detected at the 9th week of gestational development, glucagon-positive cells at the 10th week of development, and somatostatin-positive cells at the 11th week of development. However, the cells containing pancreatic polypeptide were identified by these authors only at the 17th week of development. Differences in the timing of endocrine cell differentiation can be explained by the variability in the antibody clones used in these studies or individual variability [9].

It should be noted that the co-expression of several hormones occurs in the endocrine cells of the developing human pancreas. Some researchers believe that these cells may be the precursor cells of endocrine cells in the human pancreas. The localisation of cells expressing several hormones in single cells and small clusters indicates that they are present in forming islets [8]. Jensen et al. [49] and Kaligin et al. [50] found common multihormonal progenitor cells of α- and β-cells, which later differentiate into α- and β-cells, synthesising the corresponding hormones. Some of these cells remain within the duct epithelium, but most of them are located in islets in the early postnatal period. However, most authors note that there are very few of these cells [8, 40].

Data on the formation of human pancreatic islets are also controversial. In human studies on prenatal ontogenesis [8, 51–56], various forms of the cytoarchitectural organisation of the endocrine pancreas were identified: single endocrine cells, small endocrine cell clusters, as well as mantle, bipolar, and mixed islets (see above). On this basis, numerous schemes of islet morphogenesis during prenatal human development have been presented. However, there is still no consensus regarding either the number of endocrine pancreas structure forms or the time of their formation in ontogenesis.

In the study by Robb [53], the following stages of islet morphogenesis were identified: (1) formation of islet buds (10–14 weeks), (2) endocrine cell clusters with a capillary in the centre (10–16 weeks), (3) bipolar islets (after 16 weeks), (4) islets of the mantle type (after 20 weeks), and finally (5) mature islets (after 30 weeks). According to van Assche and Aerts [54], the first stage starts only at 16 weeks. In a study by von Dorsche et al. [55], islet morphogenesis was divided into three stages during human prenatal ontogeny. The first phase (14–16 weeks) is characterised by the formation of islet buds. During the second phase (17–20 weeks), islet buds separate from the ducts with the formation of mantle islets. During the third phase (21–26 weeks), mosaic islets are formed.

In the work by Jeon et al. [8], clusters containing several types of endocrine cells were found in the pancreas at 12 weeks of development. Between weeks 8 and 11, the distribution of endocrine cells was scattered, but by week 12, insulin- and/or glucagon-producing cells started to form small clusters; by week 14, these clusters were more prominent, with a core of insulin-positive cells surrounded by glucagon-positive cells, i.e. mantle islets. By weeks 16–17, the ring of glucagon-positive cells surrounding the core of insulin-positive cells appeared to 'open up', and, later, insulin- and glucagon-positive cells had expanded and formed homogeneous insulin-secreting and glucagon-secreting cell clusters.

In our studies, we examined pancreatic autopsies derived from human foetuses from the 10th to the 40th weeks of gestational development, using histological, IHC, and morphometric methods. To analyse the dynamics of pancreatic endocrine cell quantity, we used the classification in which the foetal period of human development can be divided into four subperiods (pre-foetal, 10–12 gestational weeks (g.w.); early foetal, 13–20 g.w.; mid-foetal, 21–28 g.w.; and late foetal, 29–40 g.w.) [44].

The spatio-temporal distribution of various structural forms of endocrine pancreas in general coincides with what has been described in the literature [8, 40, 41, 44, 48, 51, 57]. However, the data obtained in our study allowed us to clarify the main stages of the morphogenesis of the endocrine part of the pancreas during prenatal human development.

In the prefoetal period, only single pancreatic endocrine cells and their small clusters were detected. Starting from 10 g.w., insulin-, glucagon-, and somatostatin-containing cells were identified within primary ducts of the human pancreas. Mantle islets were detected starting from 12 weeks. The diameter of the mantle islets was approximately 70 microns. In prenatal human development, so-called bipolar islets were also identified (β-cells located at one islet pole and α- and δ-cells at the other pole). These bipolar islets were identified starting from 14 weeks. The average diameter of bipolar islets was more than 80 microns. The largest bipolar islets were detected during the early foetal period; their diameter gradually decreased after this point. In adults, bipolar islets are not detected. Currently, the role of bipolar islets in the formation of the endocrine pancreas is not clear. According to some literature data, homogeneous clusters consisting of only β- or α-cells are present in the human foetal pancreas [8, 51]. In our study, large homogeneous clusters of endocrine cells in close contact with each other were also found. However, during the analyses of serial sections, it was shown that these clusters are parts of bipolar islets. Thus, islets consisting of only one type of endocrine cell are artefacts of two-dimensional images. The typical adult mixed islets appear in the mid-foetal period (after 25 weeks); their number gradually increases until birth. The diameter of these islets exceeds 100 microns. This 'mosaic' (mixed) islet formation seems to be related to the migration processes of different types of endocrine cells within islets.

Thus, various morphological forms of organisation of the endocrine pancreas appear consistently during human pancreas development (**Figure 2**). The first endocrine cells are detected in the central ducts of the developing human pancreas. At later stages of development, the largest pancreatic islets are also located in the central region, around the main pancreatic duct, which corresponds to literature data [8, 48]. During endocrine pancreas development, heterochronous maturation occurs, which may represent a physiological reserve for adaptation to increased metabolic load during this time.

It is important to note that all detected forms of endocrine pancreas organisation are described in pancreas phylogenesis. The chronology of the appearance of various forms of the human endocrine pancreas during ontogenesis repeats the phylogenetic stages of islet formation [58].

In normal physiological development, the ratio of various structural forms of the endocrine pancreas changes: the number of small islets and clusters of endocrine cells with a diameter of 40 to 55 microns gradually decreases, while the number of medium-sized (with a diameter of 55 to 100 microns) and large-sized (with a diameter of over 100 microns) islets increases.

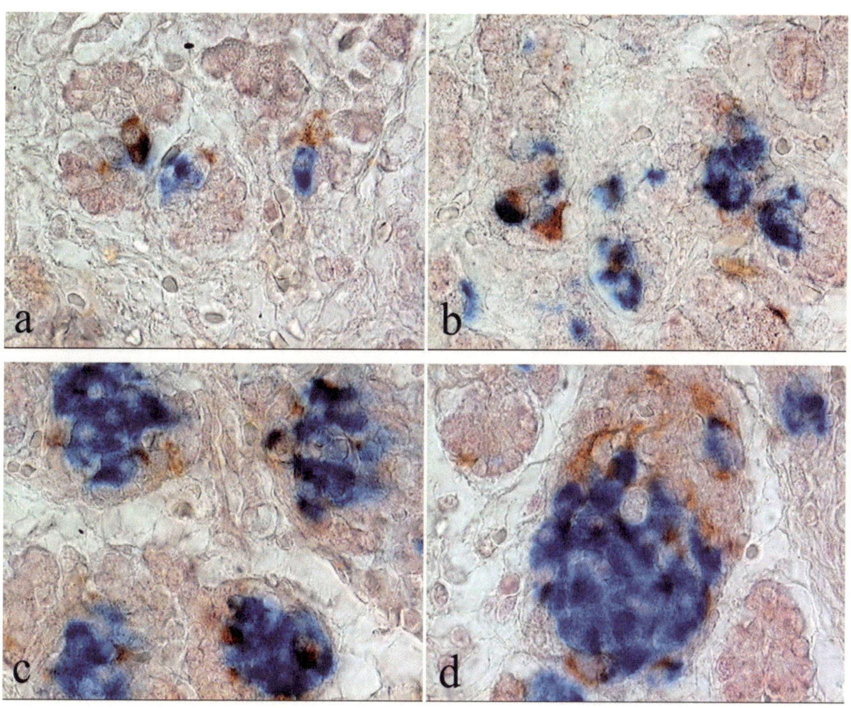

Figure 2.
Forms of endocrine pancreas structural organisation in the human foetus at 22 w.p.c.: (a) single endocrine cell, (b) small cluster of endocrine cells, (c) islet of mantle type, and (d) bipolar islet. Double immunohistochemical labelling with antibodies to glucagon (red) and insulin (blue), objective x100.

Another important issue is the timing of the appearance of mature endocrine cells, similar to those observed in adults. von Dorsche et al. [47, 55] suggested that islet β-cells start to function at 10–14 weeks. In a study by Piper et al. [40], it was shown that endocrine cells are in contact with CD34-positive cells of developing capillaries from the 10th week of development and a thin capillary islet network forms at the 14th week. According to Piper et al. [40], this is evidence of the similarity of pancreatic islets at 12–14 weeks of development with adult islets. Islet innervation starts at 12 weeks. Moreover, so-called neuro-insular complexes may be detected in the developing human pancreas starting at this time [59]. However, Jeon et al. [8] have shown that large pancreatic islets of the mixed type, typical in adults, are formed only after 21 weeks of development. In studies by Meier et al. [35] and Gregg et al. [36], the islets of Langerhans, typical in adults, were formed only at 2 years of age. This was accompanied by an increase in the number of β-cells. Thus, there is an increase in the ratio of β-cells to α-cells, as well as an increase in the ratio of β-cells to δ-cells, both due to an increase in β-cell proliferation and a decrease in the number of δ-cells [36]. The β-cell proliferation index is highest during the first 2 years after birth and then gradually decreases [35, 36].

In general, since the appearance of the first endocrine cells at 9–10 weeks of gestational development and up to 2 years of age, there is a gradual shift towards the predominance of mixed islets, but this prevalence is not complete [8, 35, 36, 53].

Modern ideas about the formation of the human endocrine pancreas are mostly limited to the primary stages of differentiation of endocrine cells and the formation of mantle islets, similar in structure to rodent islets (i.e. the period from 9 to 14 gestational weeks). Although the formation of mantle-type islets in rodents is well described, the formation of mixed islets in the developing human pancreas has been insufficiently studied [8, 9].

4. Transcription control of gene specification during pancreas ontogeny

A good model for studying the differentiation of pancreatic cells is the study of transcription factors, which play an important role in development. As described above, pancreatic endocrine cells are of endodermal origin and differentiate during prenatal development from the epithelial cells of the primary ducts. A specific programme of transcription factor gene expression is subsequently activated and defines the fate of pancreatic progenitors [60]. Through intense research over the last several years, a hierarchy of transcription factors regulating pancreas development has emerged. The expression of the same transcription factors as in mice and rats was found in human pancreatic samples using IHC methods, in situ hybridisation, and molecular biology methods (RT-qPCR, microarray). For some transcription factors, the dynamics of changes in expression levels were revealed during pancreas development [8, 40, 61, 62].

Early markers of emerging pancreatic cells include two transcription factors: pancreatic and duodenal homeobox 1 (Pdx 1) and pancreas-specific transcription factor 1a (Ptf1a). In mice, the initial expression of Pdx1 (E8.5–E9.0) marks the pre-pancreatic endoderm before it has visibly thickened. Early Pdx1 expression is therefore a useful marker of pancreatic identity, although it expands over the next several days of development to encompass the posterior stomach, duodenum, and bile duct. Although early pancreas buds still form, Pdx1 knockout mice show completely arrested pancreas organogenesis after the initial stages. Lineage tracing analysis has revealed the contribution of Pdx1-positive cells to all adult pancreatic fates. In the adult pancreas, Pdx1 is most highly expressed in β-cells and δ-cells, with lower expression in exocrine cells [7]. In humans, Pdx1 has been detected in cell nuclei at the inception of pancreatic bud outgrowth from the duodenum at 26 d.p.c. [40]. Pdx1 detection was initially accompanied by very weak detection of SOX9 in the presumptive pancreatic endoderm [62]. This expression was much more robustly detected in all pancreatic epithelial cells at 41 d.p.c. and during the early foetal period. Following islet formation, Pdx1 remained in the nuclei of non-endocrine epithelial cells. However, a more diffuse pattern of staining was observed in islet cells, consisting of both cytoplasmic and nuclear detections. By dual immunofluorescence at 14 w.p.c., this expression colocalised strongly with insulin. Later, during human foetal development and in adult pancreatic sections, Pdx1 expression remained in duct cells but was most strongly detected in islets, in keeping with its established role in glucose-regulated insulin production [40]. According to Jeon et al. [8], IHC analyses showed that IPF1, the human homologue of Pdx1, is expressed in epithelial progenitor cells throughout the period from 7 to 21 weeks, as well as in insulin-expressing cells as they appear. However, IPF1 expression was also observed in occasional glucagon-expressing cells at early but not at later stages of development. The expression of IPF1 in glucagon-expressing cells was weaker than that observed in pancreatic progenitor cells or in insulin-expressing cells. In the absence of Pdx1 expression, pancreas aplasia has been observed, with impaired growth of the dorsal diverticulum [63, 64]. Haploinsufficiency of IPF1 leads to maturity onset diabetes of the young (MODY4), an autosomal dominant form of diabetes caused by monogenic mutations [64]. Recent reports further emphasise the important role of Pdx1 in β-cell formation and function. Thus, Pdx1 plays essential roles in both pancreas development and adult islet function [7].

Another transcription factor, Ptf1a, is also expressed in the early pancreas, and its endodermal expression remains pancreas-specific throughout development. Ptf1a expression is necessary for exocrine differentiation [65], as well as endocrine cells [66]. In the absence of Ptf1a expression, the differentiation of exocrine cell precursors into duodenal cells has been observed, as well as the localisation of a small number of endocrine cells in the spleen. Consistent with its later phase of expression, Ptf1a has been identified as an acinar gene activator, and Ptf1a-deficient pancreata entirely lack acinar cells [67]. Thus, the expression of these factors plays crucial roles in pancreas specification and is necessary for normal pancreas development.

The transitions of Pdx1 and Ptf1a expression coincide with the overall conversion of progenitors into mature endocrine and exocrine cells. This conversion is also reflected in the dynamic expression of the transcription factor neurogenin 3 (Neurog3, also known as Ngn3), which specifically marks precursors of all endocrine pancreas cells [49, 67–69]. Ngn3 is a basic helix-loop-helix protein and marks the progenitor population of cells fated to form the endocrine lineage. Animals lacking Ngn3 are devoid of islets and die shortly after birth due to hyperglycaemia [68]. Within the embryonic pancreas, Ngn3 expression peaks at embryonic day 15.5, shortly after the secondary transition that indicates the burst of endocrine specification, and subsequently declines. Ngn3+ cells appear in small numbers in the early organ [7]. Expression of Ngn3 peaks by the end of the first trimester and disappears at about the 35th week of gestation [70]. Probably, similar to neurons, islet cells are ordinarily generated during a restricted developmental window [67]. In general, ectopic expression of Ngn3 causes cells to exit from the cell cycle and to express some endocrine markers [71]. Inactivation of Ngn3 leads to the failure of pancreatic islet development [68]. However, it is clear that mere overexpression of Ngn3 does not guarantee expansion into the β-cell lineage. In fact, in the majority of studies, increased glucagon- or somatostatin-expressing cells are observed [69].

In contrast to published data from mouse embryos, during human pancreas development, Jennings et al. [62] detected only a single phase of Ngn3 expression and endocrine differentiation from approximately 8 weeks, before which Nirenberg and Kim homeobox 2.2 (NKX2.2) was not observed in the pancreatic progenitor cell population. The expression of Ngn3 has been detected in the human pancreas at the 7th week of development. By the 9th week of development, the expression level of this transcription factor gradually increases and remains high until the 17th week, after which it gradually decreases [8]. Most authors have paid special attention to cells that co-express transcription factors and hormones of endocrine cells of the pancreas [61], considering these cells to be a population of progenitor cells. In the early (8–11) weeks of gestation of the human foetal pancreas, cells co-expressing Ngn3 and Pdx1, Ngn3 and insulin, and Ngn3 and glucagon have been observed.

Ngn3 controls the expression of a number of other islet-specific transcription factors, i.e. NeuroD1, Pax4, and Pax6. During pancreas development, NeuroD1 also takes part in the differentiation of endocrine cells and the morphogenesis of pancreatic islets. A reduction in the number of endocrine cells, especially β-cells, and the inability to form islets were shown in neonatal mice missing a functionally active NeuroD1 gene [72]. Unlike Ngn3+ precursors, cells expressing NeuroD1 do not proliferate (they leave the cell cycle before the activation of NeuroD1 expression) [49]. Pax4 is necessary for the differentiation of β- and δ-cells from Ngn3+ precursors, and Arx is required for the differentiation of α- and PP-cells from Ngn3+ precursors. These two transcription factors have the opposite effect (they inhibit each other) and regulate the ratio of various types of endocrine cells. In the absence of Pax4 expression (Pax4−/−), β- and δ- cells are not detected in islets [73]. In the absence of Arx expression (Arx−/−), islets are composed only of β- and δ-cells [74]. Pax6 is expressed in all types of endocrine cells; cells expressing Pax6 differentiate into α-cells, and cells simultaneously expressing Pax6 and Pax4 differentiate into β-, δ-, and PP-cells [74]. Inactivation of Pax6 leads to a decrease in the number of endocrine cells, especially α-cells, and the disorganisation of pancreatic islets [75]. Inactivation of Pax6 and Pax4 simultaneously leads to the absence of endocrine cells.

The expression of Pax4 (a marker of β-cell precursors) begins at the 9th week of human development, and the expression of Arx (a marker of α-cell precursors) begins at the 11th week [8] . Transcription factors (Nkx2–2 and Nkx6–1) play a regulatory role in the development of the endocrine part of the pancreas. The absence of Nkx6–1 expression in deficient mice leads to impaired β-cell differentiation [76]. In mice lacking Nkx2–2, there is a lack of β-cells and a decrease in the number of α-cells and PP-cells [77]. A number of transcription factors that are expressed during the differentiation of endocrine cells of the pancreas are also characteristic of the differentiation of nervous system cells [49, 68, 69, 71, 72, 78, 79]. Expression Nkx2.2 and Nkx6.1 has been detected in the human pancreas from week 7 of development, gradually increasing from week 7 to week 21 [8].

Thus, the use of transcription factors allows us to estimate the direction and features of differentiation of cellular populations in the pancreas. Data on the localisation of cells expressing various transcription factors in the developing human pancreas are few. It is important to note that, in the adult human pancreas, the maintenance of β-cell identity is associated with the presence of key transcription factors (in particular PDX1 and NKX6.1) and changes in their expression and/or localisation have been described in the islets of type 2 diabetic individuals, possibly contributing to β-cell dedifferentiation (i.e. the regression to a progenitor-like state) in this disease [70].

In our studies we have analysed the distribution of two transcription factors—NeuroD1 and Nkx6.1—in the developing human pancreas. The study was performed on pancreatic samples from 22 foetuses (gestational age 10–36-37 weeks) using double and triple immunohistochemistry with antibodies to NeuroD1 (mouse monoclonal; Abcam), Nkx6.1 (rabbit polyclonal; Thermo Fisher Scientific, Inc.), insulin (mouse monoclonal, Sigma), and glucagon (mouse monoclonal, Sigma, or rabbit polyclonal; Thermo Fisher Scientific, Inc.). Reactions of double immunohistochemical labelling were visualised using the MultiVision Polymer Detection System Anti-Rabbit HRP + Anti-Mouse AP, LV blue and LV Red (Thermo Fisher Scientific, Inc.) according to specification. In the reactions of triple immunohistochemical labelling, at the first phase, NeuroD1 was visualised using UltraVision ONE Detection System, DAB Plus Chromogen (Thermo Fisher Scientific, Inc.). At the second phase, insulin and glucagon were visualised using MultiVision Polymer Detection System Anti-Rabbit HRP + Anti-Mouse AP, LV blue and LV Red (Thermo Fisher Scientific, Inc.).

In agreement with the literature [8, 61], we showed that NeuroD1 and Nkx6.1 are present in the foetal pancreas already at 8 w.p.c. (10th g.w.). In the prefoetal period (10–12 g.w.), immunopositive reaction to NeuroD1 and Nkx6.1 was detected in the nuclei of single epithelial cells of primitive ducts (**Figures 3a** and **4a**). At these stages, the intensity of the reaction to both NeuroD1 and Nkx6.1 was very low. The reaction to these transcription factors became more intensive by the beginning of the early foetal period (14 g.w.) (**Figures 3b** and **4b**) and remains high in all subsequent stages of development. The same results demonstrating that the expression level of NeuroD1 was initially low and increases starting from week 15 onwards and the expression of Nkx6.1 gradually increases from the 7th to the 21st weeks of development were shown by other authors [8].

As it was previously shown, in the pancreas of foetuses from 8 to 21 weeks of development, NeuroD1 is colocalised with insulin, glucagon, somatostatin, and pancreatic polypeptide indicating the involvement of this transcription factor in the differentiation of all four types of endocrine cells [61]. At the same time, positive reaction to Nkx6.1 was detected only in the insulin-containing cells, suggesting that Nkx6.1 is β-cell-specific transcription factor.

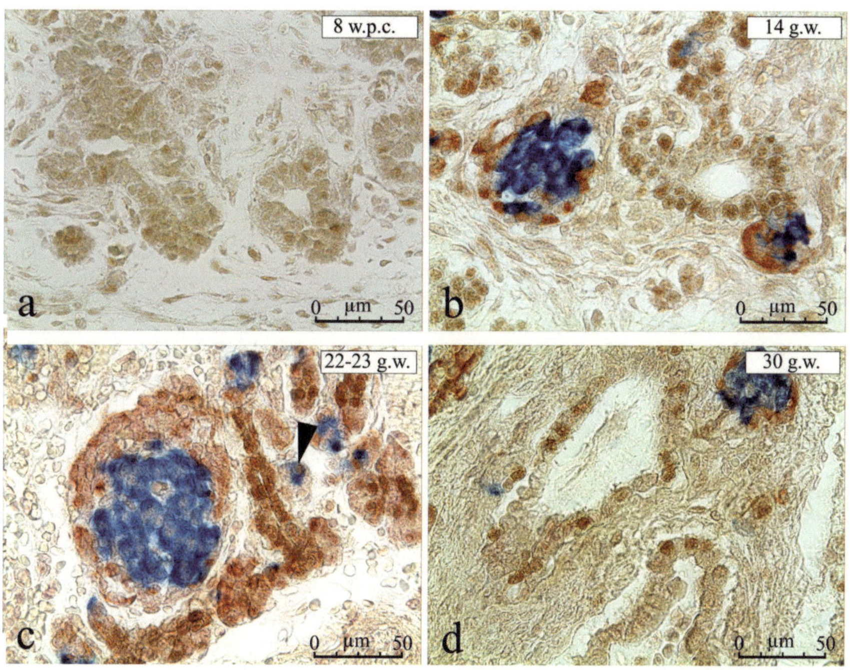

Figure 3.
Distribution of the transcription factor NeuroD1 in the human foetal pancreas. (a) Immunohistochemical staining to NeuroD1 in the foetal pancreas at 8 w.p.c. (b–d): triple immunohistochemical staining to NeuroD1 (brown nuclei), insulin (blue), and glucagon (red) in the foetal pancreas at 14 g.w. (b), 22–23 g.w. (c), and 30 g.w. (d). Arrowhead indicates β-cell with NeuroD1-positive nucleus.

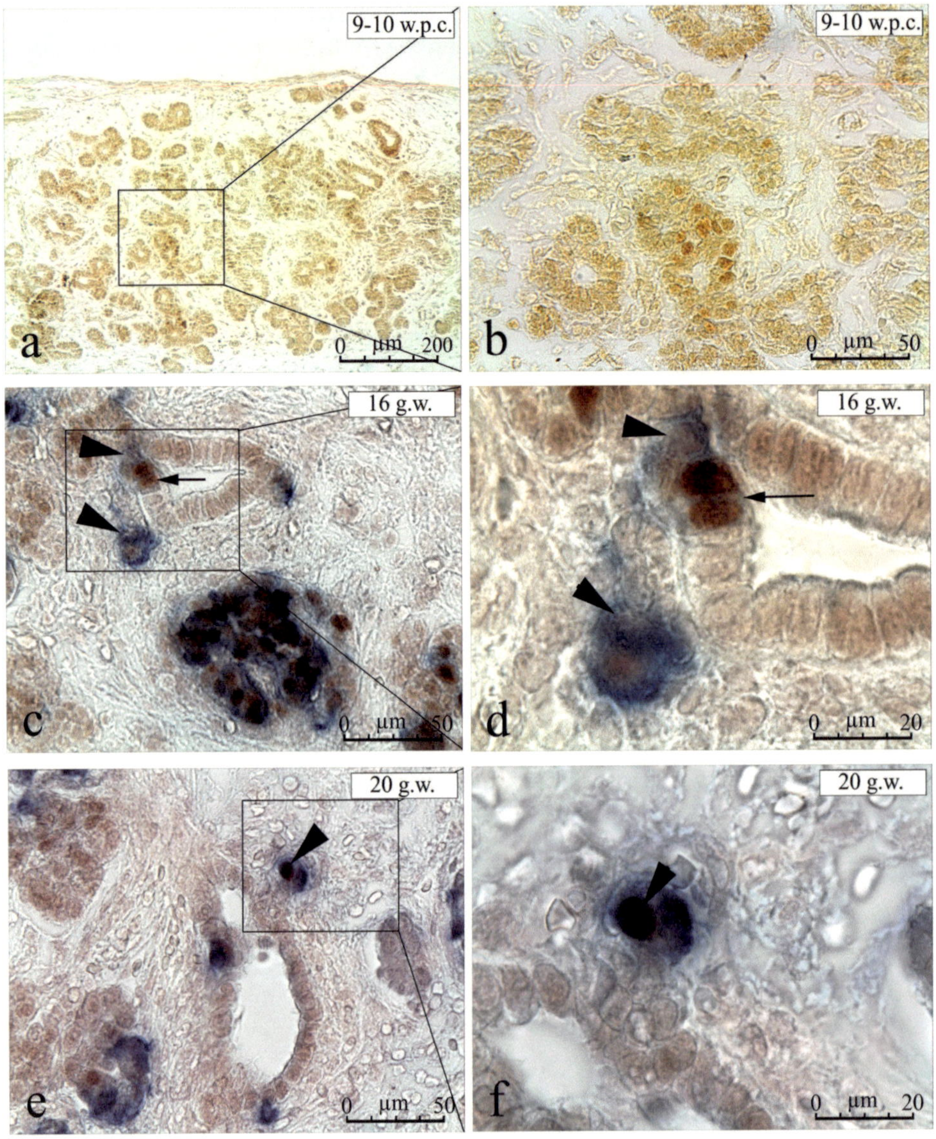

Figure 4.
Distribution of the transcription factor Nkx6.1 in the human foetal pancreas. (a, b) Immunohistochemical staining to Nkx6.1 in the foetal pancreas at 9–10 w.p.c. and (c, d) double immunohistochemical staining to Nkx6.1 (brown) and insulin (blue) in the fetal pancreas at 16 g.w.; arrowheads indicate β-cells with Nkx6.1-negative nuclei; arrows indicate hormone-negative cells with Nkx6.1-positive nuclei. e, f - double immunohistochemical staining to Nkx6.1 (brown) and glucagon (blue) in the fetal pancreas at 20 g.w.; arrowheads indicate α-cells with Nkx6.1-positive nucleus. b, d and f – marked fragments of a, c and e at higher magnification.

Our findings demonstrate that the distribution of NeuroD1 and Nkx6.1 in the developing human pancreas was different. The amount of NeuroD1-positive cells gradually increases during prefoetal period, and, in the early and middle foetal periods, such cells were more numerous. Starting from 14th g.w. onwards, positive reaction to NeuroD1 was observed predominantly in the epithelial ductal cells (**Figure 3b–d**). In the majority of endocrine islet cells, the reaction to NeuroD1 was immunonegative. However, in all investigated pancreatic samples, we found single β- and α-cells with NeuroD1-positive nuclei (**Figure 3c**), which is in agreement with the literature [61]. In the late foetal period, NeuroD1 is also expressed predominantly in the epithelial ductal cells, but the distribution of NeuroD1-positive cells became sparser (**Figure 3d**).

Starting from the beginning of early foetal period (14 g.w.) and in all subsequent stages of development, positive reaction to Nkx6.1 was observed predominantly in insulin-containing β-cells (**Figure 4c–f**) which indicates the involvement of Nkx6.1 in β-cell differentiation. In all investigated pancreatic samples, we observed two types of β-cells: β-cells with the Nkx6.1-positive nuclei which represent the majority of β-cells and rare population of β-cells with the Nkx6.1-immunonegative nuclei (**Figure 4c,d**). In addition, in the pancreas of all foetuses from 14th to 36–37th g.w., we identified hormone-negative cells with Nkx6.1-positive nuclei (**Figure 4c,d**). It can be suggested that Nkx6.1 is transiently expressed in the differentiating β-cells prior to hormone synthesis, and then its expression decreases and is further restored in the mature β-cells. On the other hand, differentiation of some β-cells may occur without Nkx6.1 expression. As it was shown in mice lacking Nkx6.1 (Nkx6.1−/−) expression, Nkx6.1 does not affect the early stages of pancreas development and β-cell differentiation [76]. The defect in Nkx6.1 expression appears after E12.5 and results in the significant reduction of the amount of β-cells (up to 85% of wild type) and in the absence of the expression of the mature β-cell markers MAFA and Glut2 [76, 78].

In contrast to other researchers [61], we found rare glucagon-containing cells with Nkx6.1-positive nuclei in the developing human pancreas (**Figure 4e, f**). Activation of Nkx6.1 expression in α-cells has been previously observed in a mouse model after extreme β-cell loss [17] and in humans with type 1 diabetes [80]. This activation of Nkx6.1 possibly indicates α- to β-cell conversion during restoration of β-cell mass [17] or a partial change of α-cells towards a β-cell phenotype [80].

5. Conclusions

This chapter has provided a brief analysis of the current state of research in the field of the origin of pancreatic endocrine cell populations and islet growth. However, further research must be performed to deepen our understanding of these processes, due to their fundamental importance in the restoration of normal glucose homeostasis in humans with impaired carbohydrate metabolism.

Acknowledgements

This work was supported by the Russian Foundation for Basic Research, Project №. 18-015-00147.

Conflict of interest

The authors declare no competing interests.

Author details

Alexandra E. Proshchina[1*], Yuliya S. Krivova[1], Larisa E. Gurevich[2], Valeriy M. Barabanov[1], Dmitriy A. Otlyga[1], Iya A. Voronkova[3] and Sergey V. Saveliev[1]

1 Research Institute of Human Morphology, Moscow, Russia

2 Moscow Regional Clinical Research Institute n.a. M.F. Vladimirskiy, Moscow, Russia

3 Endocrinology Research Centre, Moscow, Russia

*Address all correspondence to: proshchina@yandex.ru

References

[1] IDF Diabetes Atlas. 6th ed. Brussels: International Diabetes Federation; 2013. 159 p

[2] Karam JH, Grodsky GM, Forsham PH. Insulin secretion in obesity: Pseudodiabetes? The American Journal of Clinical Nutrition. 1968;**21**(12):1445-1454. DOI: 10.1093/ajcn/21.12.1445

[3] Bonner-Weir S. Regulation of pancreatic beta-cell mass in vivo. Recent Progress in Hormone Research. 1994;**49**:91-104. DOI: 10.1016/b978-0-12-571149-4.50008-8

[4] Bernard-Kargar C, Ktorza A. Endocrine pancreas plasticity under physiological and pathological conditions. Diabetes. 2001;**50**(1):S30-S35. DOI: 10.2337/diabetes.50.2007.s30

[5] Bonner-Weir S. Beta-cell turnover: Its assessment and implications. Diabetes. 2001;**50**(Suppl 1):S20-S24. DOI: 10.2337/diabetes.50.2007.s20

[6] Chhabra P, Kensinger CD, Moore DJ, Brayman KL. Present accomplishments and future prospects of cell-based therapies for type 1 diabetes mellitus. In: Wagner D, editor. Type 1 Diabetes - Pathogenesis, Genetics and Immunotherapy. Shanghai: InTech; 2011. pp. 295-335. DOI: 10.5772/22343

[7] Puri S, Hebrok M. Cellular plasticity within the pancreas— Lessons learned from development. Developmental Cell. 2010;**18**(3):342-356. DOI: 10.1016/j.devcel.2010.02.005

[8] Jeon J, Correa-Medina M, Ricordi C, Edlund H, Diez JA. Endocrine cell clustering during human pancreas development. The Journal of Histochemistry and Cytochemistry. 2009;**57**(9):811-824. DOI: 10.1369/jhc.2009.953307

[9] Krivova YS, Proshchina AE, Barabanov VM, Saveliev SV. Development of the islets of Langerhans in the human fetal pancreas. In: Satou A, Nakamura H, editors. Pancreas: Anatomy, Diseases and Health Implications. NY: Nova Science Publishers; 2012. pp. 53-88. https://www.novapublishers.com/catalog/product_info.php?products_id=37414

[10] Bonner-Weir S, Baxter LA, Schuppin GT, Smith FE. A second pathway for regeneration of adult exocrine and endocrine pancreas. A possible recapitulation of embryonic development. Diabetes. 1993;**42**(12):1715-1720. DOI: 10.2337/diab.42.12.1715

[11] Bouwens L, Klöppel G. Islet cell neogenesis in the pancreas. Virchows Archiv. 1996;**427**(6):553-560. DOI: 10.1007/bf00202885

[12] Bouwens L, Lu WG, De Krijger R. Proliferation and differentiation in the human fetal endocrine pancreas. Diabetologia. 1997;**40**(4):398-404. DOI: 10.1007/s001250050693

[13] Bouwens L. Transdifferentiation versus stem cell hypothesis for the regeneration of islet beta-cells in the pancreas. Microscopy Research and Technique. 1998;**43**(4):332-336. DOI: 10.1002/(sici)1097-0029(19981115)43:4%3C332::aid-jemt7%3E3.0.co;2-1

[14] Yuan S, Rosenberg L, Paraskevas S, Agapitos D, Duguid WP. Transdifferentiation of human islets to pancreatic ductal cells in collagen matrix culture. Differentiation. 1996;**61**:67-75. DOI: 10.1046/j.1432-0436.1996.6110067.x

[15] Bonner-Weir S, Li WC, Ouziel-Yahalom L, Guo L, Weir GC, Sharma A. Beta-cell growth and regeneration: Replication is only part of the story. Diabetes. 2010;**59**(10):2340-2348. DOI: 10.2337/db10-0084

[16] Iaglov VV, Eletskiĭ IK. Morphology and classification of the acino-islet cells of the pancreas [article in Russian]. Arkhiv Anatomii, Gistologii i émbriologii. 1975;**69**(12):20-23

[17] Thorel F, Népote V, Avril I, Kohno K, Desgraz R, Chera S, et al. Conversion of adult pancreatic alpha-cells to beta-cells after extreme beta-cell loss. Nature. 2010;**464**(7292):1149-1154. DOI: 10.1038/nature08894

[18] Chera S, Baronnier D, Ghila L, Cigliola V, Jensen JN, Gu G, et al. Diabetes recovery by age-dependent conversion of pancreatic δ-cells into insulin producers. Nature. 2014;**514**(7523):503-507. DOI: 10.1038/nature13633

[19] Saito K, Iwama N, Takahashi T. Morphometrical analysis on topographical difference in size distribution, number and volume of islets in the human pancreas. The Tohoku Journal of Experimental Medicine. 1978;**124**:177-186. DOI: 10.1620/tjem.124.177

[20] Rahier J, Wallon J, Henquin JC. Cell populations in the endocrine pancreas of human neonates and infants. Diabetologia. 1981;**20**:540-546. DOI: 10.1007/bf00252762

[21] Wierup N, Svensson H, Mulder H, Sundler F. The ghrelin cell: A novel developmentally regulated islet cell in the human pancreas. Regulatory Peptides. 2002;**107**(1-3):63-69. DOI: 10.1016/s0167-0115(02)00067-8

[22] Wierup N, Sundler F, Heller SR. The islet ghrelin cell. Journal of Molecular Endocrinology. 2013;**52**(1):R35-R49. DOI: 10.1530/jme-13-0122

[23] Gutierrez GD, Gromada J, Sussel L. Heterogeneity of the pancreatic beta cell. Frontiers in Genetics. 2017;**8**:22. DOI: 10.3389/fgene.2017.00022

[24] Bouwens L, Pipeleers DG. Extra-insular beta cells associated with ductules are frequent in adult human pancreas. Diabetologia. 1998;**41**(6): 629-633. DOI: 1007/s001250050960

[25] Bosco D, Armanet M, Morel P, Niclauss N, Sgroi A, Muller YD, et al. Unique arrangement of α- and β-cells in human islets of Langerhans. Diabetes. 2010;**59**:1202-1210. DOI: 10.2337/db09-1177

[26] Kilimnik G, Zhao B, Jo J, Periwal V, Witkowski P, Misawa R, et al. Altered islet composition and disproportionate loss of large islets in patients with type 2 diabetes. PLoS One. 2011;**6**(11):e27445. DOI: 10.1371/journal.pone.0027445

[27] Atkinson MA, Maclaren NK. Perspectives islet cell autoantigens in insulin-dependent diabetes. The Journal of Clinical Investigation. 1993;**92**(10):1608-1616. DOI: 10.1172/jci116745

[28] Kim A, Miller K, Jo J, Wojcik P, Hara M. Islet architecture – A comparative study. Islets. 2009;**1**:129-136. DOI: 10.4161/isl.1.2.9480

[29] Kilimnik G, Jo J, Periwal V, Zielinski MC, Hara M. Quantification of islet size and architecture. Islets. 2012;**4**:167-172. DOI: 10.4161/isl.19256

[30] Ku S, Lee H, Lee J. An immunohistochemical study on the pancreatic endocrine cells of the C57BL/6 mouse. Journal of Veterinary Science. 2002;**3**(4):327-333

[31] Cabrera O, Berman DM, Kenyon NS, Ricordi C, Berggren P, Caicedo A. The unique cytoarchitecture of human pancreatic islets has implications for islet cell function. Proceedings of the National Academy of Sciences of the United States of America. 2006;**103**(7):2334-2339. DOI: 10.1073/pnas.0510790103

[32] Brissova M, Flower MJ, Nicholson WE, Chu A, Hirshberg B, Harlan DM,

et al. Assessment of human pancreatic islet architecture and composition by laser scanning confocal microscopy. The Journal of Histochemistry and Cytochemistry. 2005;**53**(9):1087-1097. DOI: 10.1369/jhc.5c6684.2005

[33] Proshchina AE, Savel'yev SV. Immunohistochemical study of α- and β-cell distribution in human pancreatic Langerhans islets of various types. Bulletin of Experimental Biology and Medicine. 2013;**155**(6):798-801. DOI: 10.1007/s10517-013-2255-5

[34] Barbieux C, Parnaud G, Lavallard V, Brioudes E, Meyer J, Alibashe Ahmed M, et al. Asymmetrical distribution of δ and PP cells in human pancreatic islets. Journal of Endocrinology. 2016;**229**(2):123-132. DOI: 10.1530/JOE-15-0542

[35] Meier JJ, Butler AE, Saisho Y, Monchamp T, Galasso R, Bhushan A, et al. Beta-cell replication is the primary mechanism subserving the postnatal expansion of beta-cell mass in humans. Diabetes. 2008;**57**:1584-1594. DOI: 10.2337/db07-1369

[36] Gregg BE, Moore PC, Demozay D, Hall BA, Li M, Husain A, et al. Formation of a human β-cell population within pancreatic islets is set early in life. The Journal of Clinical Endocrinology and Metabolism. 2012;**97**(9):3197-3206. DOI: 10.1210/jc.2012-1206

[37] Winer S, Tsui H, Lau A, Song A, Li X, Cheung RK, et al. Autoimmune islet destruction in spontaneous type 1 diabetes is not β-cell exclusive. Nature Medicine. 2003;**9**:198-205. DOI: 10.1038/nm818

[38] Rodriguez-Diaz R, Abdulreda MH, Formoso AL, Gans I, Ricordi C, Berggren P, et al. Innervation patterns of autonomic axons in the human endocrine pancreas. Cell Metabolism. 2011;**14**(1):45-54. DOI: 10.1016/j.cmet.2011.05.008

[39] Lee I. Human pancreatic islets develop through fusion of distinct β and α/δ islets. Development, Growth & Differentiation. 2016;**58**:635-640. DOI: 10.1111/dgd.12308

[40] Piper K, Brickwood S, Turnpenny LW, Cameron IT, Ball SG, Wilson DI, et al. Beta cell differentiation during early human pancreas development. The Journal of Endocrinology. 2004;**181**: 11-23. DOI: 10.1677/joe.0.1810011

[41] Pan FC, Brissova M. Pancreas development in humans. Current Opinion in Endocrinology, Diabetes, and Obesity. 2014;**21**(2):77-82. DOI: 10.1097/MED.0000000000000047

[42] Dolenšek J, Pohorec V, Rupnik MS, Stožer A. Pancreas physiology. In: Seicean A, editor. Challenges in Pancreatic Pathology. Rijeka, Croatia: IntechOpen; 2017. pp. 19-52. DOI: 10.5572/65895

[43] Riopel M, Li J, Fellows GF, Goodyer CG, Wang R. Ultrastructural and immunohistochemical analysis of the 8-20 week human fetal pancreas. Islets. 2014;(4):e982949. DOI: 10.4161/19382014.2014.982949

[44] Milvanov AP, Saveliev SV. Rational periodization of prenatal human development and methodical aspects of embryology. In: Milvanov AP, Saveliev SV, editors. Prenatal Human Development. [in Russian]. Moscow, Russia: MDV; 2006. pp. 21-32

[45] Boĭko IG, Prokopchik NI. Age-related morphometric characteristics of the human pancreas [article in Russian]. Arkhiv Anatomii, Gistologii i émbriologii. 1987;**93**(12):79-81

[46] Meier JJ, Köhler CU, Alkhatib B, Sergi C, Junker T, Klein HH, et al. Beta-cell development and turnover during prenatal life in humans. European Journal of Endocrinology. 2010;**162**: 559-568. DOI: 10.1530/eje-09-1053

[47] von Dorsche HH, Falkmer S. Ontogeny of human Langergans islets. A review of some light- and electron-microscopical, immunogistochemikal and functional data on fetal development of the endocrine pancreas. Journal of Physiology and Biochemistry. 2000;**36**(6):701-718

[48] Polak M, Bouchareb-Banaei L, Scharfmann R, Czernichow P. Early pattern of differentiation in the human pancreas. Diabetes. 2000;**49**(2):225-232. DOI: 10.2337/diabetes.49.2.225

[49] Jensen J, Heller RS, Funder-Nielsen T, Pedersen EE, Lindsell C, Weinmaster G, et al. Independent development of pancreatic α- and β-cells from neurogenin3-expressing precursors. A role of the notch pathway in repression of premature differentiation. Diabetes. 2000;**49**(2):163-176. DOI: 10.2337/diabetes.49.2.163

[50] Kaligin MS, Gumerova AA, Titova MA, Andreeva DI, Sharipova ÉI, Kiiasov AP. C-kit is a marker of human pancreatic endocrinocyte stem cells [article in Russian]. Morfologiia. 2011;**140**(4):32-37

[51] Falin LI. The development and cytodifferentiation of the islets of Langerhans in human embryos and foetuses. Acta Anatomica (Basel). 1967;**68**(1):147-168. DOI: 10.1159/000143023

[52] Ferner H. Das Inselsystem Des Pankreas: Entwicklung, Histobiologie Und Pathophysiologie Mit Besonderer Berucksichtigung Des Diabetes Mellitus [German]. Stuttgart: Thieme; 1952. 186 p

[53] Robb P. The development of the islets of Langerhans in the human foetus. Experimental Physiology. 1961;**46**:335-343. DOI: 10.1113/expphysiol.1961.sp001551

[54] van Assche AF, Aerts L. The fetal endocrine pancreas. Contributions to Gynecology and Obstetrics. 1979;**5**:44-57

[55] von Dorsche HH, Reiher H, Hahn FU. Phases in the early development of the human islet organ. Anatomischer Anzeiger. 1988;**166**:69-76

[56] Bocian-Sobkowska J, Zabel M, Wozniak W, Surdyk-Zasada J. Polyhormonal aspect of the endocrine cells of the human fetal pancreas. The Journal of Histochemistry and Cytochemistry. 1999;**112**(2):147-153. DOI: 10.1007/s004180050401

[57] Nair G, Hebrok M. Islet formation in mice and men: Lessons for the generation of functional insulin-producing β-cells from human pluripotent stem cells. Current Opinion in Genetics & Development. 2015;**32**:171-180. DOI: 10.1016/j.gde.2015.03.004

[58] Eletskiĭ IK, Iaglov VV. Evolution of the Structural Organization of the Vertebrate Endocrine Pancreas [in Russian]. Moscow, Russia: Nauka; 1978. 166 p

[59] Krivova YS, Proshchina AE, Barabanov VM, Saveliev SV. Neuro-insular complexes in the human pancreas. In: Seicean A, editor. Challenges in Pancreatic Pathology. Rijeka, Croatia: IntechOpen; 2017. pp. 3-17. DOI: 10.5572/65059

[60] Ben-Othman N, Courtney M, Vieira A, Pfeifer A, Druelle N, Gjernes E, et al. From pancreatic islet formation to beta-cell regeneration. Diabetes Research and Clinical Practice. 2013;**101**(1):1-9. DOI: 10.1016/j.diabres.2013.01.013

[61] Lyttle BM, Li J, Krishnamurthy M, Fellows F, Wheeler MB, Goodyer CG, et al. Transcription factor expression in the developing human fetal endocrine pancreas. Diabetologia. 2008;**51**(7):1169-1180. DOI: 10.1007/s00125-008-1006-z

[62] Jennings RE, Berry AA, Kirkwood-Wilson R, Roberts NA, Hearn T, Salisbury RJ, et al. Development of the human pancreas from foregut to endocrine commitment. Diabetes. 2013;**62**(10): 3514-3522. DOI: 10.2337/db12-1479

[63] Jonsson J, Carlsson L, Edlund T, Edlund H. Insulin-promoter-factor 1 is required for pancreas development in mice. Nature. 1994;**371**(6498):606-609. DOI: 10.1038/371606a0

[64] Stoffers DA, Zinkin NT, Stanojevic V, Clarke WL, Haberner JF. Pancreatic agenesis attributable to a single nucleotide deletion in the human IPF1 gene coding sequence. Nature Genetics. 1997;**51**(1):106-110. DOI: 10.1038/ng0197-106

[65] Hale MA, Kagami H, Shi L, Holland AM, Elasser HP, Hammer RE, et al. The homeodomain protein PDX1 is required at mid-pancreatic development for the formation of exocrine pancreas. Developmental Biology. 2005;**286**(1):225-237. DOI: 10.1016/j.ydbio.2005.07.026

[66] Kawaguchi Y, Cooper B, Gannon M, Ray M, Macdonald RJ, Wright CV. The role of the transcriptional regulator Ptf1a in converting intestinal to pancreatic progenitors. Nature Genetics. 2002;**32**(1):128-134. DOI: 10.1038/ng959

[67] Murtaugh LC. Pancreas and beta-cell development: From the actual to the possible. Development. 2007;**134**(3):427-438. DOI: 10.1242/dev.02770

[68] Gradwohl G, Deirich A, LeMeur M, Guillemot F. Neurogenin3 is required for the development of the four endocrine cell lineages of the pancreas. Proceedings of the National Academy of Sciences of the United States of America. 2000;**97**(4):1607-1611. DOI: 10.1073/pnas.97.4.1607

[69] Schwitzgebel VM, Scheel DW, Conners JR, Kalamaras J, Lee JE, Anderson DJ, et al. Expression of neurogenin3 reveals an islet cell precursor population in the pancreas. Development. 2000;**127**:3533-3542

[70] Marchetti P, Bugliani M, De Tata V, Mara S, Marselli L. Pancreatic beta cell identity in humans and the role of type 2 diabetes. Frontiers in Cell and Development Biology. 2017;**5**:55. DOI: 10.3389/fcell.2017.00055

[71] Apelqvist A, Li H, Sommer L, Beatus P, Anderson DJ, Honjo T, et al. Notch signalling controls pancreatic cell differentiation. Nature. 1999;**400**(6747):877-881. DOI: 10.1038/23716

[72] Naya FJ, Huang H, Qui Y, Muton H, Demayo FJ, Leiter AB, et al. Diabetes, defective pancreatic morphogenesis, and abnormal enteroendocrine differentiation in BETA2/NeuroDdeficient mice. Genes & Development. 1997;**11**(18):2323-2334. DOI: 10.1101/gad.11.18.2323

[73] Sosa-Pineda B, Chowdhury K, Torres M, Oliver G, Gruss P. The Pax4 gene is essential for differentiation of insulin-producing beta cells in the mammalian pancreas. Nature. 1997;**386**(6623):406-409. DOI: 10.1038/386399a0

[74] Collombat P, Mansouri A, Hecksher-Sorensen J, Serup P, Krull J, Gradwohl G, et al. Opposing actions of Arx and Pax4 in endocrine pancreas development. Genes & Development. 2003;**17**(20):2591-2603. DOI: 10.1101/gad.269003

[75] Ashery-Padan R, Zhou X, Marquardt T, Herrera P, Toube L, Berry A, et al. Conditional inactivation of Pax6 in the pancreas causes early onset of diabetes. Developmental Biology. 2004;**269**(2):479-488. DOI: 10.1016/j.ydbio.2004.01.040

[76] Sander M, Sussel L, Conners J, Scheel D, Kalamaras J, Dela Cruz F, et al.

Homeobox gene Nkx6.1 lies downstream of Nkx2.2 in the major pathway of β-cell formation in the pancreas. Development. 2000;**127**(24):5533-5540

[77] Jorgensen MC, Ahnfelt-Ronne J, Hald J, Madsen O, Serup P, Hecksher-Sorensen J. An illustrated review of early pancreas development in the mouse. Endocrine Reviews. 2007;**28**(6):685-705. DOI: 10.1210/er.2007-0016

[78] Henseleit KD, Nelson SB, Kuhlbrodt K, Hennings CJ, Ericson J, Sander M. NKX6 transcription factor activity is required for α- and β-cell development in the pancreas. Development and Disease. 2005;**132**(13):3139-3149. DOI: 10.1242/dev.01875

[79] Bonal C, Herrera PL. Genes controlling pancreas ontogen. The International Journal of Developmental Biology. 2008;**52**(7):823-835. DOI: 10.1387/ijdb.072444cb

[80] Brissova M, Haliyur R, Saunders D, Shrestha S, Dai C, Blodgett DM, et al. α cell function and gene expression are compromised in type 1 diabetes. Cell Reports. 2018;**22**(10):2667-2676. DOI: 10.1016/j.celrep.2018.02.032

Chapter 3

Deltamethrin Alters Thyroid Hormones and Delays Pubertal Development in Male and Female Rats

Shui-Yuan Lu, Pinpin Lin, Wei-Ren Tsai and Chen-Yi Weng

Abstract

Pyrethroid insecticides are suspected endocrine-disrupting chemicals. Deltamethrin has been reported to antagonize thyroid hormone receptor activity in a reporter assay. We hypothesized that deltamethrin alters thyroid function. Male and female rats were administered daily oral gavages with 0, 0.3, 1, or 3 mg/kg/day deltamethrin on postnatal days 23–53 and 22–42, respectively. Results showed that deltamethrin decreased the relative thyroid weight in 0.3 and 1 mg/kg/day in female but not in male rats. Although the histology and several parameters of thyroid were not affected, the decreased relative weight exhibited underlying meaning. Deltamethrin delayed the age of vaginal opening (VO) and increased body weight upon VO in 3 mg/kg/day. Deltamethrin failed to delay the age of preputial separation in male rats. In the respective of serum hormone concentration, deltamethrin increased 17β-estradiol (E_2) with dose-dependent manner in female rats. The novel finding is that deltamethrin decreased thyroxine (T_4), triiodothyronine (T_3), and thyroid-stimulating hormone (TSH) in the female rats. In contrast, deltamethrin increased T_3 and TSH but not in T_4 in male rats. We inferred that deltamethrin disrupts thyroid hormone and might be related to estrogen receptor agonist. The future work is to investigate if deltamethrin disrupts the hypothalamus-pituitary-thyroid axis.

Keywords: thyroid hormone, deltamethrin, vaginal opening, preputial separation, pubertal rats

1. Introduction

Environmental endocrine disruptors (EDs) have been the subject of public attention since the publication of Rachel Carson's Silent Spring [1]. Problems associated with EDs have been studied, and EDs have been suggested not only to produce reproductive and developmental toxicity in experimental animals but also to increase the incidence of cancers, such as those of the mammary gland, testis, and prostate, and to decrease sperm numbers and induce developmental abnormalities in wildlife and humans by disrupting the endocrine system [2, 3]. Faced with an emerging health threat, the U.S. Environmental Protection Agency (U.S. EPA) identified research requirements for future risk assessments regarding endocrine-disrupting chemicals (EDCs) [4, 5].

The Endocrine Disruptor Screening and Testing Advisory Committee of the U.S. EPA has recommended a screening strategy to investigate endocrine-disrupting compounds that are agonists/antagonists to estrogen/androgen receptors, steroid biosynthesis inhibitors, or altering thyroid hormone function [6]. Pubertal female and male rat models were designed to investigate alterations of female and male pubertal development, thyroid function, and hypothalamic-pituitary-thyroid (HPT) function, respectively. The intact 22- or 23-day-old weanling female and male rats were exposed to the test substance for 20 or 30 days during the pubertal development period [7, 8].

HPT function has been used extensively to review vertebrate species, teleosts, amphibians [9, 10], and mammals [11, 12]. In normal thyroid gland functioning, thyrotropin-releasing hormone (TRH) is released from the hypothalamus. TRH travels to the anterior pituitary and triggers the release of thyroid-stimulating hormone (TSH), or thyrotropin, from the thyrotrophic cells in the pars distalis of the adenohypophysis. An increase in TSH production leads to an increase in thyroid hormone (TH) synthesis. TSH binds to receptors on the membrane of the thyroid follicle cells, thereby stimulating the biosynthesis of the iodine-containing THs, thyroxine (T4), and triiodothyronine (T3). T4 is the principle TH secreted from the thyroid gland; however, it is quickly metabolized into T3, the more potent TH. T3 and T4 can exert negative feedback control over anterior pituitary to inhibit further release of TSH [13, 14].

Synthetic pyrethroids are a class of insecticides listed by the U.S. EPA as potential EDCs [15]. Pyrethroids are widely used in agriculture and public health. Deltamethrin ((S)-α-cyano-3-phenoxybenzyl-(1R)-cis-(2, 2-dibromovinyl)-2, 2-dimethylcyclo-propane carboxylate) is the membrane of the type-II synthetic pyrethroid pesticide, which is commonly used worldwide. The major site of action of deltamethrin seems to be the voltage-dependent sodium channel. However, most recent studies on deltamethrin-related toxicity have focused on testicular and epididymal toxicity with decreasing weights, damage to the diameter of seminiferous tubules [16], abnormal morphology of spermatozoa, and sloughing and vacuolization [17–23] in male rats and mice. The second related form of toxicity caused by deltamethrin is neurotoxicity. Previous studies have shown that deltamethrin-induced neurobehavioral toxicity [24] in parent rats and increased cytochrome P450 expression are involved in the neuroendocrine functions in their offspring [25, 26]. The most significant effects of neurotoxicity in rats include decreased neuronal sodium channel expression [27, 28], motor coordination deficit [29], decreased motor activity and activity of the striatal dopaminergic system [30], cell death in the hippocampus and deficits in hippocampal precursor proliferation [31], and decreased ambulatory motor activity [32]. A previous study showed that deltamethrin decreases messenger RNA expression of specific genes that may potentially disrupt normal adipogenesis and lipid and glucose metabolism [33]. Recently, an epidemiologic finding showed that deltamethrin might be a risk factor for attention deficit hyperactivity disorder [34].

Although deltamethrin induces male reproductive toxicity and neurotoxicity, it remains unclear whether deltamethrin causes endocrine disruption. According to structural similarities and in vitro research, pyrethroid insecticides (including deltamethrin and its metabolite, 3-phenoxybenzoic acid) can affect the TH system by interfering with the nuclear TH receptors [35]. Furthermore, daily administration of 6.25–25 mg/kg/day deltamethrin for 15 days was shown to decrease the serum and cerebral cortex levels of T4 and T3 in the mitochondria of the cortex and hippocampi of rats [36]. However, in another study, an oral gavage with a single 15 mg/kg dose of deltamethrin or 3 mg/kg/day of deltamethrin for 30 days failed to change TH levels [37].

However, the exposure time for the high dosage (15 mg/kg) may have been too short, and when a lower dosage (3 mg/kg/day for 30 days) was administered, exposure may have been too low to disturb TH levels. Little is known about the molecular and cellular mechanisms that mediate TH action in the developing brain or developmental events [38].

The Toxicology in the 21st Century (Tox21) program is a federal collaboration between U.S. government agencies. The program utilizes high-throughput screening (HTS) to quickly and efficiently test chemicals for activity across a battery of assays targeting cellular processes such as the agonistic and antagonistic activities of androgen receptors, estrogen receptors, and thyroid receptors (TRs) [39]. The Tox21 databank showed that deltamethrin exhibited TR antagonistic activity. Furthermore, Du et al. [35] showed that deltamethrin exhibited TR and androgen receptor antagonistic activities in reporter assays. Few studies have investigated endocrine-disrupting activity in nuclear receptors (especially in androgen receptors, estrogen receptors, and TRs) or deltamethrin-induced dysfunction of the hypothalamus-pituitary-gonad (HPG) and HPT axes; many studies, however, have investigated male reproductive toxicity and neurotoxicity. Based on previous reports regarding testicular and epididymal toxicity, neurotoxicity, and TR receptor antagonists from the Tox21 databank, we hypothesized that deltamethrin might disturb thyroid-related function. We studied pubertal development and thyroid function in male and female Wistar rats to investigate the possible effects of deltamethrin on endocrine activity [35].

2. Materials and methods

2.1 Chemicals

The following materials were obtained: testosterone propionate (TP, purity ≥ 97%), flutamide (purity ≥ 97%), corn oil (0.9 g/ml), 17α-ethinylestradiol (purity ≥ 98%) (Sigma-Aldrich Co., St. Louis, MO, USA), and deltamethrin (purity ≥ 97%; Sinon Co., Taichung, Taiwan, ROC).

2.2 Animals

The animal use protocol was reviewed and approved by the Institutional Animal Care and Use Committee of the Taiwan Agricultural Chemicals and Toxic Substances Research Institute. Five-week-old male and female Wistar rats were purchased from BioLASCO (Taipei, Taiwan, ROC). The rats were acclimated to the laboratory environment and reared under a controlled temperature (21 ± 2°C), humidity (40–70%), frequency of ventilation (at least 10/h), and alternating 12 h cycles of light and darkness. The rats were administered a pellet rodent diet and water ad libitum until they were sacrificed. At 12 weeks of age, the 18 male and 18 female rats within each treatment group were allowed to mate over a 14-day period. Gestation day (GD) 0 was defined as the day that sperm was observed in the vagina of the female following mating. Dams were allowed to deliver their pups naturally. Any litters with fewer than eight pups (i.e., including both male and female pups) or not delivered by GD 23 were excluded from the study. Sufficient litter numbers needed to be available to assure that 7–10 female and 10 male pups were available per treatment group and to avoid the need for placing littermates in the same experimental groups. A population of female and male pups that was as homogeneous as possible was selected by eliminating an equal number of pups from the heavy and the light ends of the distribution, leaving the number of animals required in the middle of the distribution. The pups were assigned to treatment groups such that the mean body weights and variances for all groups were similar. Animal allocation to treatment groups was conducted on the basis of body weight randomization to ensure unbiased weight distribution across all groups.

2.3 Treatment

Each male offspring was weighed and clinically observed, and measurements were recorded daily prior to treatment. Treatments (control; TP 0.4 mg/kg/day; flutamide 3 mg/kg/day; deltamethrin 0.3, 1, or 3 mg/kg/day) were administered daily by oral gavage on postnatal day (PND) 23–53. Beginning on PND 30, males were examined daily for preputial separation (PPS). Males were dosed and sacrificed from 2 h after dosing on PND 53. Each female offspring was weighed and clinically observed, and its measurements were recorded daily prior to treatment. Treatments (control; 17α-ethinyl estradiol [EE] 5 mg/kg/day; deltamethrin 0.3, 1, or 3 mg/kg/day) were administered daily by oral gavage from PND 22 to 42. Females were examined daily for vaginal opening (VO). Females were dosed and sacrificed from 2 hours after dosing on PND 42.

2.4 Clinical signs and body weights

Throughout the study period, each female and male animal was observed at least once daily for clinical signs of toxicity related to chemical treatment. On working days, all cages were checked in the mornings and afternoons for dead or moribund animals. The body weight of each rat was recorded to the nearest 0.1 g daily prior to treatment.

2.5 Measurement of organ weights

Twenty-four hours after the final treatment, each rat was treated with the control (females and males); EE 5 mg/kg/day (females); TP 0.4 mg/kg/day (males); flutamide 3 mg/kg/day (males); and deltamethrin 0.3 or 1 mg/kg/day (females and males) and anesthetized with Zoletil 3 mg/kg/day (females and males) in the same sequence that the test substance was administered. Uteri and ovaries were dissected and carefully trimmed of fat to avoid loss of luminal content. The body of each uterus was cut just above its junction with the cervix and at the junction of the uterine horns with the ovaries. Each uterus was weighed with and without the luminal content. Thyroids, livers, kidneys, pituitary glands, adrenal glands, ovaries, seminal vesicles, and coagulating glands with and without fluid, prostates, levator ani plus bulbocavernosus muscles (LABC), epididymides, testes, and penes were carefully dissected and weighed.

2.6 VO

Each female animal was examined daily for VO from PND 21. On the day that VO was first detected, the age and body weight were recorded. Vaginal lavage was collected daily from the day following VO until the end of the study by repeated pipetting of 0.9% saline into the vagina. The lavage fluid was applied to a clean glass slide, and the smear was viewed immediately under low magnification (×100) with a microscope. Cytology was evaluated and the stage of the estrous cycle was determined using the method described by Everett [40]. The appearance of a small "pinhole," vaginal thread, and complete VO were all recorded on the days they were observed. The day of complete VO was the endpoint in the analysis for the age upon VO; a pinhole or thread did not represent complete VO, even though it had to be recorded when observed. However, if any animal within any treatment group showed incomplete opening (such as persistent threads or a pinhole) for more than 3 days, a separate analysis was conducted using the ages at which an incomplete opening was first observed. Even if VO otherwise appeared complete, documentation of a vaginal thread was crucial. It was also critical that the "initiation" of VO be recorded and preferred that VO observations be taken daily after dosing. Whether collected before or after dosing, VO observations had to be collected at approximately the same time each day.

2.7 Estrous cyclicity

From the day of VO up to and including the day of necropsy, daily vaginal smears were obtained and evaluated under a low-power light microscope for the presence of leukocytes, nucleated epithelial cells, or cornified epithelial cells. The vaginal smears were classified as diestrus (predominance of leukocytes mixed with some cornified epithelial cells), proestrus (predominance of clumps of round, nucleated epithelial cells), or estrus (predominance of cornified epithelial cells), and the stages were recorded daily. Metestrus was classified as an early part of diestrus rather than a late part of estrus. Age upon first vaginal estrus was noted, and it was preferred (although not critical) that estrous cycle observations be made after daily dosing. Whether collected before or after dosing, estrous cycle observations had to be collected at approximately the same time each day.

At the end of the study, the overall pattern of each female was characterized as regularly cycling (having recurring 4- to 5-day cycles), irregularly cycling (having cycles with periods of diestrus longer than 3 days or periods of cornification longer than 2 days), or not cycling (having prolonged periods of either vaginal cornification or leukocytic smears). In cases where there were too few days between VO and the end of the study for more than one cycle to be observed, classification was based on the available data with the default assumption that the animals cycled regularly if the partial data fit the definition and irregularly if the study ended without being able to distinguish between irregular cycling and not cycling.

2.8 PPS

PPS, the separation of the foreskin of the penis from the glans, is an early reliable marker of the pubertal progression that normally occurs between 40 and 50 days of age, with an average of 43 days, depending on the rat species [41]. In the present study, PPS was monitored from PND 22 to 53. All males were monitored at approximately the same time each day. A partial separation with a thread of cartilage remaining was recorded as partial, but only the day of complete separation was used in the data analysis. The appearance of partial and complete PPS or a persistent thread of tissue between the glans and prepuce were all recorded on the days they were observed. The day of complete PPS was the endpoint used in the analysis for the age upon PPS. However, if any animal in any treatment group showed incomplete separation (including persistent threads) for more than 3 days, a separate analysis was conducted using the ages at which partial separation was first observed. Even if PPS otherwise appeared complete, documentation of a thread was crucial. It was also critical that "initiation" of PPS be recorded and preferred that PPS observations be taken after daily dosing. Whether collected before or after dosing, the PPS observations had to be collected at approximately the same time each day.

2.9 Hematochemistry

Blood samples treated with control (females and males), EE 5 mg/kg/day (females), TP 0.4 mg/kg/day (males), flutamide 3 mg/kg/day (males), and deltamethrin 0.3, 1, and 3 mg/kg/day (female and male) were collected and coagulated for 30 min in an SST II tube (#367953, BD Co., Plymouth, UK). The blood samples were put on ice bath prior to centrifugation. After coagulation, the blood was centrifuged at 3000 × *g* for 15 min. The serum was transferred into siliconized microcentrifuge tubes and stored at −80°C until used. Serum creatinine and blood urea nitrogen levels were detected with an automated clinical chemistry analyzer (DRI-CHEM 4000i, Fujifilm Co., Tokyo, Japan).

2.10 Hormonal measurements

Luteinizing hormone (LH); follicle-stimulating hormone (FSH); T4, T3, and TSH levels in serum treated with control (females and males); EE 5 mg/kg/day (females); TP 0.4 mg/kg/day (males); flutamide 3 mg/kg/day; and deltamethrin 0.3, 1, and 3 mg/kg/day (females and males) were determined using a magnetic bead panel (#RPTMAG-86K, #PTHYMAG-30K, Millipore Co., St. Charles, MI, USA).

Testosterone (T) and estradiol (E2) levels in serum treated with control (female and male), 5 mg/kg/day 17α-ethinyl estradiol (EE 5) (female), 0.4 mg/kg/day testosterone propionate (TP 0.4) (male), 3 mg/kg/day flutamide, 0.3, 1, and 3 mg/kg/day deltamethrin (female and male) were assayed using EIA kit (#582701, #582251, Cayman Co.). Luteinizing hormone (LH), follicle-stimulating hormone (FSH), total tetraiodothyronine (T4), triiodothyronine (T3), and thyroid-stimulating hormone (TSH) levels in serum treated with control (female and male), 5 mg/kg/day 17α-ethinyl estradiol (EE 5) (female), 0.4 mg/kg/day testosterone propionate (TP 0.4) (male), 3 mg/kg/day flutamide, 0.3, 1, and 3 mg/kg/day deltamethrin (female and male) were determined using magnetic bead panel (#RPTMAG-86K, #PTHYMAG-30K, Millipore Co.). A cytochrome P450 19A1 ELISA kit (CSB-EL006394RA, Cusabio Co.) was used for determined aromatase level in serum treated with control (female and male), 5 mg/kg/day 17α-ethinyl estradiol (EE 5) (female), 0.4 mg/kg/day testosterone propionate (TP 0.4) (male), 3 mg/kg/day flutamide, 0.3, 1, and 3 mg/kg/day deltamethrin (female and male).

2.11 Histology

The tissues of the thyroid glands (females and males), pituitary glands (females and males); uteri, ovaries, testes, epididymides, and prostates of rats treated with control (females and males); EE 5 mg/kg/day (females); TP 0.4 mg/kg/day (males); flutamide 3 mg/kg/day; and deltamethrin 0.3, 1, and 3 mg/kg/day (females and males) were stored in 10% formaldehyde solution for at least 7 days. After routine processing, 3-μm-thick paraffin sections were cut and stained with hematoxylin and eosin. Thyroid sections were subjectively evaluated for several parameters of thyroid activity including total area analyzed (μm^2), total colloid area (μm^2), colloid/total area (%), number of colloid, average colloid area (μm^2), average colloid diameter (μm), total epithelial area (μm^2), and epithelial/total area (%) [42] by Tissue Phenomics (Definiens AG, Munich, Germany).

3. Statistical analysis

Data are expressed as the mean ± standard deviation (SD). Data for the mean initial or necropsy body weight, mean age, body weight upon VO or PPS, organ weight, and hormone levels were analyzed for homogeneity of variance by using Bartlett's test. When samples were proven to be homogeneous, nonparametric analysis of variance was applied. Absolute organ weight was analyzed using analysis of covariance with body weight upon necropsy as a covariate. When a significant treatment effect was observed, Dunnett's test (control vs. treatment groups) was used to compare the treatment groups. The level of statistical significance was set a priori at $\alpha = 0.05$.

4. Results

4.1 Effects on body and organ weights

During the study period, no clinical signs of toxicity were detected in any treatment group of male or female rats. EE significantly decreased the body weights of the female rats from PND 25 to 42 (**Figure 1A**). However, in contrast to the control group, deltamethrin did not change the body weight of the female or male rats (**Figure 1B**).

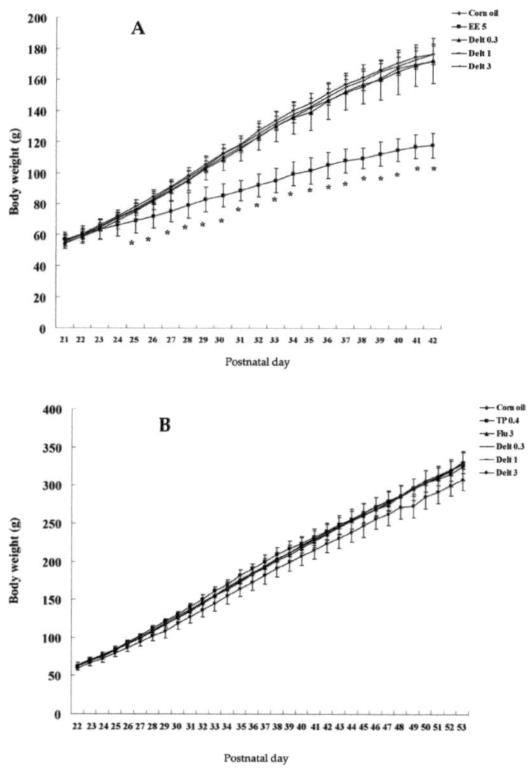

Figure 1.
*Body weight changes in Wistar female rats treated with 17α-ethinyl estradiol 5 mg/kg/day (EE5), testosterone propionate 0.4 mg/kg/day (TP 0.4), flutamide 3 mg/kg/day (Flu 3), and deltamethrin 0.3, 1, and 3 mg/kg/day (Delta 0.3, Delta 1, and Delta 3). Female rats were dosed daily starting at 21 days of age and this was continued until necropsy on day 42 (A), and male rats were dosed daily starting at 22 days of age and this was continued until necropsy on day 53 (B). EE significantly decreased the body weight during the treatment period. Data are expressed as mean ± SD of 10 animals per treatment group. *Significantly different from the vehicle control, P < 0.05.*

Treatments	Vehicle control	EE[1] (mg/kg/day)	TP[2]	Flutamide	Deltamethrin (mg/kg/day)		
		5	0.4	3	0.3	1	3
Female							
Sample size (n)	10	10			10	10	10
Initial body weight (g)	59 ± 3	60 ± 4			59 ± 4	61 ± 4	60 ± 2
Final body weight (g)	173 ± 10	119 ± 7***			173 ± 15	177 ± 6	177 ± 7
Final body weight (%)	100	69			100	102	102
Body weight gain (g)	114 ± 9	59 ± 6***			114 ± 14	116 ± 7	117 ± 7
Male							
Sample size (n)	10		10	10	10	10	10
Initial body weight (g)	69.6 ± 3.5		70 ± 3	69 ± 5	70 ± 3	71 ± 3	66 ± 4
Final body weight (g)	331 ± 18		328 ± 25	328 ± 25	328 ± 23	331 ± 14	308 ± 14**
Final body weight (%)	100		99	99	99	100	93
Body weight gain (g)	261 ± 16		260 ± 21	257 ± 21	258 ± 22	260 ± 12	242 ± 12

[1]*EE: 17α-ethinyl estradiol;* [2]*TP: testosterone propionate, p-value = *≤0.05, **≤0.01, ***≤0.005.*

Table 1.
General growth in the female and male rats.

Treatments	Vehicle control	EE[1] (mg/kg/day)	Deltamethrin (mg/kg/day)		
		5	0.3	1	3
Sample size (n)	10	10	10	10	10
Liver (g)	8.2 ± 0.6	6.1 ± 0.4***	8.0 ± 1.2	8.1 ± 0.7	8.1 ± 0.6
Kidney (g)	1.6 ± 0.2	1.2 ± 0.1***	1.6 ± 1.2	1.6 ± 0.1	1.6 ± 0.1
Pituitary (mg)	10.2 ± 1.4	15.7 ± 6.4*	10.0 ± 1.3	10.7 ± 1.8	12.1 ± 3.3
Adrenals (mg)	55.8 ± 7.0	36.8 ± 4.8***	50.9 ± 5.9	53.1 ± 5.2	52.3 ± 7.8
Ovaries (mg)	94.3 ± 14.5	59.4 ± 13.7***	90.9 ± 17.1	92.7 ± 14.5	98.5 ± 23.7
Uterus, wet (mg)	427.5 ± 191.8	583.3 ± 328.8	383.6 ± 237.8	508.6 ± 2773.6	431.7 ± 221.5
Uterus, blotted (mg)	344.5 ± 71.8	364.6 ± 58.8	303.9 ± 93.5	357.4 ± 100.2	340.2 ± 86.6
Thyroid w/o trachea (mg)	138.3 ± 10.0	113.0 ± 12.1***	130.5 ± 10.2	135.8 ± 8.7	140.5 ± 11.9
Thyroid w/o trachea (mg)	43.4 ± 7.8	38.3 ± 5.3	36.3 ± 6.4*	36.4 ± 6.6	42.5 ± 5.1

[1]*EE: 17α-ethinyl estradiol; propionate, p-value = *≤0.05, **≤0.01, ***≤0.005.*

Table 2.
Organ weight at necropsy in the female rats.

In the female rats, EE significantly decreased final body weight and weight gain in female rats, while deltamethrin did not. In the male rats, TP, flutamide, and deltamethrin did not affect the body weight and weight gain except 3 mg/kg/day deltamethrin (**Table 1**). EE significantly changed the weights of the livers, kidneys, pituitary glands, adrenal glands, ovaries, and thyroid with trachea. For absolute organ weight treatment with 0.3 mg/kg/day, deltamethrin significantly reduced 16% of thyroid weight in the female rats, and the reduction was not dose-dependent (**Table 2**). For relative organ weight, EE significantly increased relative thyroid weight, while 0.3 and 1 mg/kg/day deltamethrin significantly decreased it (**Figure 2A**) in female rats but not in male rats (**Figure 2B**).

In the male rats, TP significantly increased the absolute organ weights of the adrenals, seminal vesicles plus coagulating glands with and without fluid, left and right epididymides, and left and right testes. Flutamide significantly decreased the absolute organ weights of the seminal vesicles plus coagulating glands, LABC, epididymides, and penes. Treatment with 3 mg/kg/day deltamethrin significantly decreased the weights of the thyroids, livers, and penes in male rats. Although treatment with 3 mg/kg/day deltamethrin significantly reduced 13% of penis weight in the male rats, the reduction was not dose-dependent (**Table 3**).

4.2 Effects on BUN, creatinine in serum

In order to investigate the effect of deltamethrin on blood chemistry, the blood urea nitrogen (BUN) and creatinine were selected as indicators. EE significantly increased BUN, while deltamethrin did not affect BUN and creatinine in female rats. TP and flutamide did affect the BUN and creatinine, while deltamethrin decreased marginally serum BUN in male rats (**Table 4**).

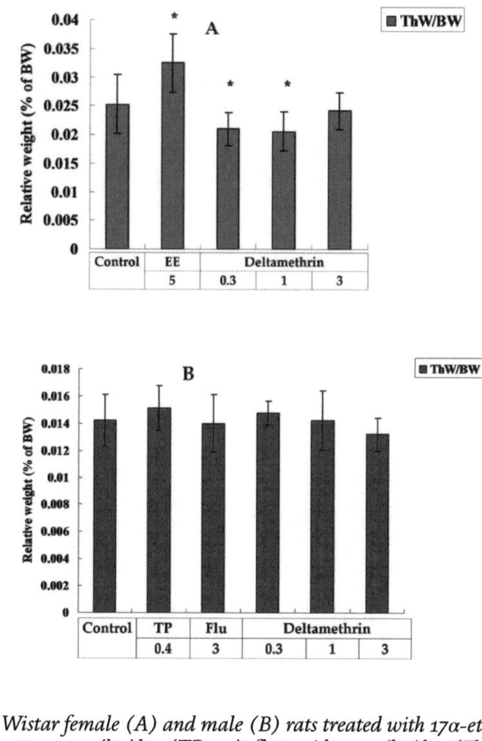

Figure 2.
*Relative thyroid weight in Wistar female (A) and male (B) rats treated with 17α-ethinyl estradiol 5 mg/kg/day (EE5), testosterone propionate 0.4 mg/kg/day (TP 0.4), flutamide 3 mg/kg/day (Flu 3), and deltamethrin 0.3, 1, and 3 mg/kg/day (Delta 0.3, Delta 1, and Delta 3). EE significantly increased relative thyroid weight, while deltamethrin in low and middle dose significantly decreased it. There is no significant difference of relative thyroid weight between control and positive, negative and deltamethrin treatments. Data are expressed as mean ± SD of 10 animals per treatment group. *Significantly different from the vehicle control, $P < 0.05$.*

Treatments	Vehicle control	TP[1]	Flutamide	Deltamethrin		
		0.4	3	0.3	1	3
Sample size (n)	10	10	10	10	10	10
Liver (g)	15.7 ± 1.1	14.8 ± 1.4	15.2 ± 1.0	14.8 ± 1.4	15.2 ± 0.8	13.6 ± 0.8***
Kidney (g)	2.7 ± 0.2	2.6 ± 0.3	2.5 ± 0.2	2.6 ± 0.2	2.6 ± 0.2	2.5 ± 0.2
Pituitary (mg)	13.3 ± 1.1	13.4 ± 1.6	13.4 ± 2.3	12.9 ± 2.2	13.1 ± 1.1	12.2 ± 1.7
Adrenals (mg)	57.5 ± 4.8	67.8 ± 5.8***	58.2 ± 7.0	56.9 ± 6.5	58.4 ± 6.0	55.5 ± 5.5
Seminal vesicle + coagulating gland, with fluid (mg)	859 ± 100	1050 ± 111***	627 ± 120***	956 ± 151	954 ± 124	852 ± 103
Seminal vesicle + coagulating gland, without fluid (mg)	540 ± 46	675 ± 109**	447 ± 67**	574 ± 68	599 ± 85	571 ± 77
Prostate (mg)	233 ± 47	255 ± 53	210 ± 57	246 ± 26	233 ± 37	218 ± 45
LABC[2] (mg)	732 ± 109	779 ± 99	585 ± 97**	733 ± 94	716 ± 82	648 ± 75
Left epididymis (mg)	229 ± 14	199 ± 10***	196 ± 24**	241 ± 20	236 ± 28	224 ± 16
Right epididymis (mg)	235 ± 21	197 ± 10***	196 ± 24**	247 ± 21	234 ± 28	217 ± 18
Left testis (mg)	1409 ± 75	1013 ± 209***	1415 ± 118	1410 ± 115	1380 ± 105	1394 ± 116
Right testis (mg)	1407 ± 59	1018 ± 218***	1432 ± 139	1388 ± 110	1409 ± 99	1390 ± 134
Thyroid with trachea (mg)	183.4 ± 23.8	188.8 ± 18.2	182.1 ± 12.4	190.3 ± 15.7	191.7 ± 12.4	175.1 ± 11.4
Thyroid without trachea (mg)	47.0 ± 7.7	49.1 ± 5.6	45.7 ± 5.8	48.5 ± 5.3	46.9 ± 6.3	40.6 ± 3.7*
Penis (mg)	253 ± 24	268 ± 19	228 ± 26*	256 ± 24	252 ± 17	234 ± 16*

[1]TP: testosterone propionate, [2]LABC: levator ani plus bulbocarvernosus muscles, p-value = $^{*}\leq 0.05$, $^{**}\leq 0.01$, $^{***}\leq 0.005$.

Table 3.
Organ weight at necropsy in the male rats.

Treatments	Vehicle control	EE[1] (mg/kg/day)	TP[2] (mg/kg/day)	Flutamide (mg/kg/day)	Deltamethrin (mg/kg/day)		
		5	0.4	3	0.3	1	3
Female							
Sample size (n)	10	10			10	10	10
BUN[3] (mg/dL)	19.1 ± 4.0	24.2 ± 3.4**			18.0 ± 2.0	17.0 ± 4.7	16.8 ± 4.4
Creatinine (mg/dL)	0.27 ± 0.05	0.24 ± 0.05			0.26 ± 0.05	0.23 ± 0.05	0.25 ± 0.05
Male							
Sample size (n)	10		10	10	10	10	10
BUN (mg/dL)	19.1 ± 2.2		19.2 ± 2.2	18.1 ± 1.9	17.5 ± 2.0	16.8 ± 2.2*	16.2 ± 2.2*
Creatinine (mg/dL)	0.29 ± 0.03		0.27 ± 0.08	0.28 ± 0.04	0.28 ± 0.04	0.3 ± 0.00	0.26 ± 0.05

*[1]EE: 17α-ethinyl estradiol; [2]TP: testosterone propionate; [3]BUN: blood urea nitrogen; p-value = *≤0.05 , **≤0.01.*

Table 4.
BUN, creatine in the female and male rats.

4.3 Effects on VO and estrous cyclicity in female rats

The mean age and body weight upon VO were 27.9 days and 95.5 g, respectively, in the control female rats. Treatment with EE significantly advanced VO to 25.4 days of age and substantially reduced the mean body weight at the time of VO to 70.7 g. VO in EE-treated rats was first detected at 24 days of age in most rats. Treatment with 3 mg/kg/day deltamethrin significantly delayed the mean time of VO (32.3 days) and increased the mean body weight to 127.3 g at the time of VO (**Figure 3A**).

The estrous cycles of individual animals were evaluated from the day after VO until the end of the study. Most control rats exhibited regular cycling, although three

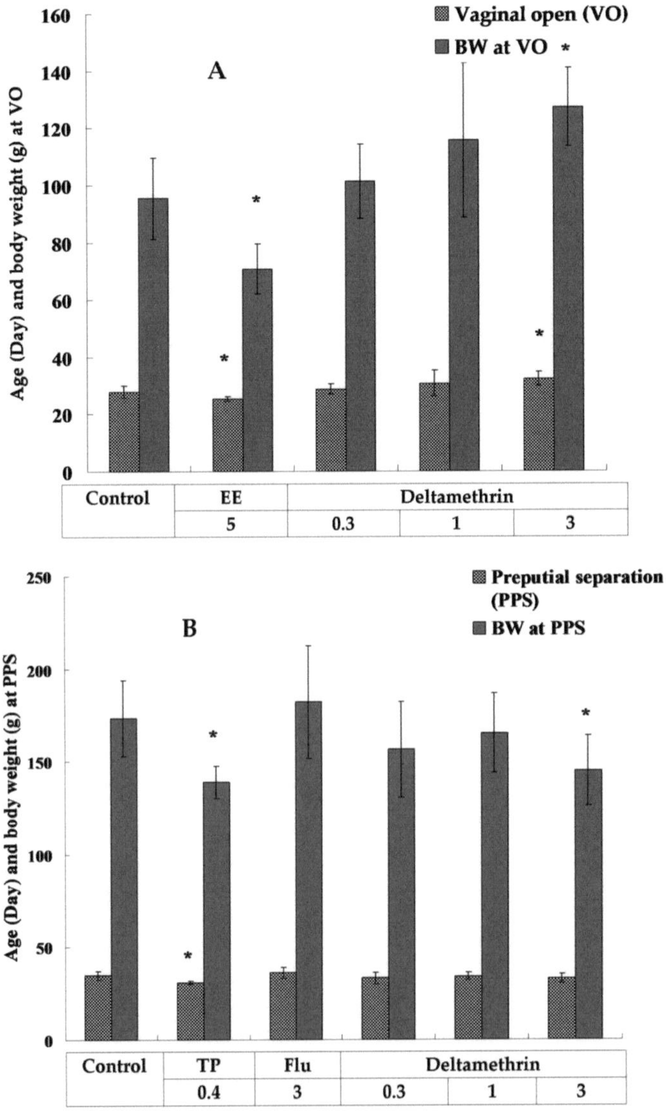

Figure 3.
*Mean age and body weight at vaginal opening (VO) in Wistar female (A) and male (B) rats treated with 17α-ethinyl estradiol 5 mg/kg/day (EE5) testosterone propionate 0.4 mg/kg/day (TP 0.4), flutamide 3 mg/kg/day (Flu 3), and deltamethrin 0.3, 1, and 3 mg/kg/day (Delta 0.3, Delta 1, and Delta 3). Animals were dosed daily starting at 21 days of age and examined from the time and body weight of vaginal opening for 21 days for female rats. Animals were dosed daily starting at 22 days of age and examined from the time and body weight of preputial separation (PPS) for 31 days for male rats. *Significantly different from the vehicle control, P < 0.05.*

Treatments	Vehicle control	EE[1] (mg/kg/day)	TP[2] (mg/kg/day)	Flutmaide (mg/kg/day)	Deltamethrin (mg/kg/day)		
		5	0.4	3	0.3	1	3
Female							
Sample size (n)	10	10			10	10	10
Total area analyzed (μm^2) ($\times 10^6$)	2.4 ± 1.1	3.6 ± 0.9			2.2 ± 0.2	2.7 ± 1.7	3.2 ± 0.6
Total colloid area (μm^2) ($\times 10^6$)	1.1 ± 0.5	1.9 ± 0.5			1.2 ± 0.2	1.2 ± 0.6	1.6 ± 0.3
Colloid/total area (%)	0.46 ± 0.04	0.51 ± 0.01			0.53 ± 0.05	0.48 ± 0.10	0.51 ± 0.06
Number of colloid	437 ± 206	869 ± 265			409 ± 16	479 ± 291	656 ± 157
Average colloid area (μm^2) ($\times 10^3$)	2.6 ± 0.2	2.2 ± 0.1			2.8 ± 0.6	2.7 ± 0.6	2.6 ± 0.9
Average colloid diameter (μm)	57.2 ± 2.3	52.5 ± 1.3			59.8 ± 6.4	58.1 ± 6.3	56.9 ± 10.3
Total epithelial area (μm^2) ($\times 10^6$)	1.2 ± 0.5	1.7 ± 0.3			0.9 ± 0.2	1.3 ± 0.9	1.5 ± 0.3
Epithelial/total area (%)	0.48 ± 0.06	0.46 ± 0.01			0.43 ± 0.07	0.47 ± 0.09	0.48 ± 0.06
Male							
Sample size (n)	10		10	10	10	10	10
Total area analyzed (μm^2) ($\times 10^6$)	4.0 ± 1.2		3.0 ± 0.7	2.8 ± 1.2	2.9 ± 0.9	3.4 ± 0.3	3.6 ± 0.4
Total colloid area (μm^2) ($\times 10^6$)	1.7 ± 0.4		1.6 ± 0.4	1.2 ± 0.5	1.4 ± 0.3	1.6 ± 0.03	1.7 ± 0.4
Colloid/total area (%)	0.44 ± 0.08		0.51 ± 0.05	0.46 ± 0.14	0.56 ± 0.07	0.47 ± 0.03	0.46 ± 0.07
Number of colloid	619 ± 304		347 ± 133	435 ± 261	515 ± 304	669 ± 80	711 ± 152
Average colloid area (μm^2) ($\times 10^3$)	2.8 ± 0.8		4.7 ± 0.8*	3.7 ± 2.6	3.2 ± 1.1	2.4 ± 0.3	2.4 ± 0.5
Average colloid diameter (μm)	59.9 ± 9.3		76.9 ± 6.8*	66.3 ± 23.2	62.7 ± 11.7	54.8 ± 3.0	55.0 ± 5.1
Total epithelial area (μm^2) ($\times 10^6$)	2.1 ± 1.0		1.4 ± 0.4	1.5 ± 0.8	1.4 ± 0.7	1.8 ± 0.3	1.8 ± 0.1
Epithelial/total area (%)	0.53 ± 0.07		0.46 ± 0.04	0.56 ± 0.13	0.48 ± 0.06	0.52 ± 0.05	0.51 ± 0.04

[1]*EE: 17α-ethinyl estradiol;* [2]*TP: testosterone propionate, p-value = *≤0.05.*

Table 5.
Measurements of several parameters of thyroid activity in treatment with deltamethrin.

rats exhibited diestrus for ≥4 days. VO occurred from PND 26 to 31. EE induced a lasting estrus in most rats and VO occurred from PND 24 to 26. Most rats treated with a low dosage (0.3 mg/kg/day) of deltamethrin had regular estrus and experienced VO from PND 26 to 32. One rat exhibited no VO. Treatment with a medium-strength dosage (1 mg/kg/day) of deltamethrin caused irregular cycling in four rats and delays in VO (PND 42) in one rat. Treatment with a high dosage (3 mg/kg/day) of deltamethrin prevented VO in two rats, irregular cycling in one rat, and a delay in VO between PND 30 and 36 in eight rats (data not shown).

4.4 Effects on PPS in male rats

The mean age and body weight of the male control rats upon PPS were 34.8 days and 173.5 g, respectively. TP substantially advanced the mean age of PPS to 30.8 days

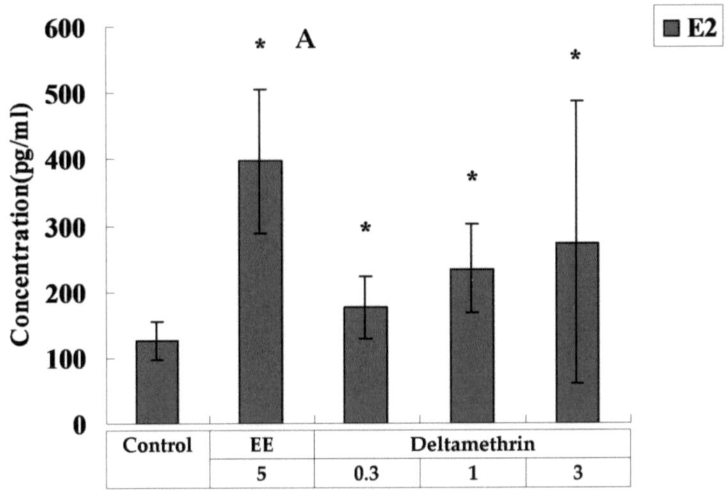

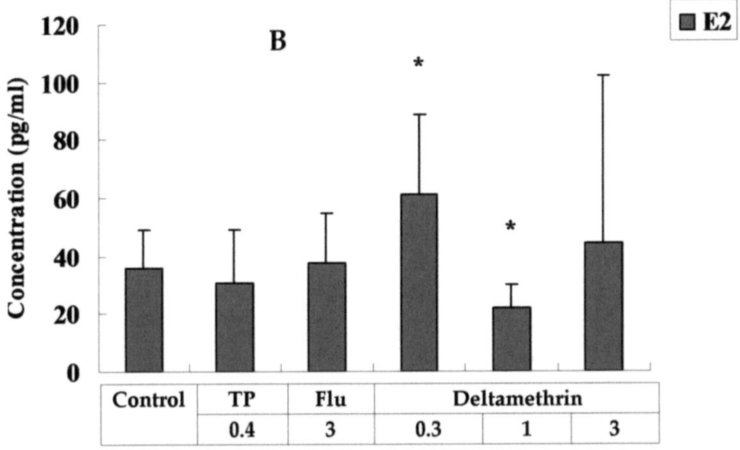

Figure 4.
Measurements of serum 17β-estradiol (E2) treated with control, 17α-ethinyl estradiol 5 mg/kg/day (EE5) testosterone propionate 0.4 mg/kg/day (TP 0.4), flutamide 3 mg/kg/day (Flu 3), and deltamethrin 0.3, 1, and 3 mg/kg/day (Delta 0.3, Delta 1, and Delta 3) in rats. EE significantly increased serum E2 concentration, while deltamethrin decreased it in female rats (A). Deltamethrin significantly increased E2 in low dose but decreased it in middle dose in male rats (B).

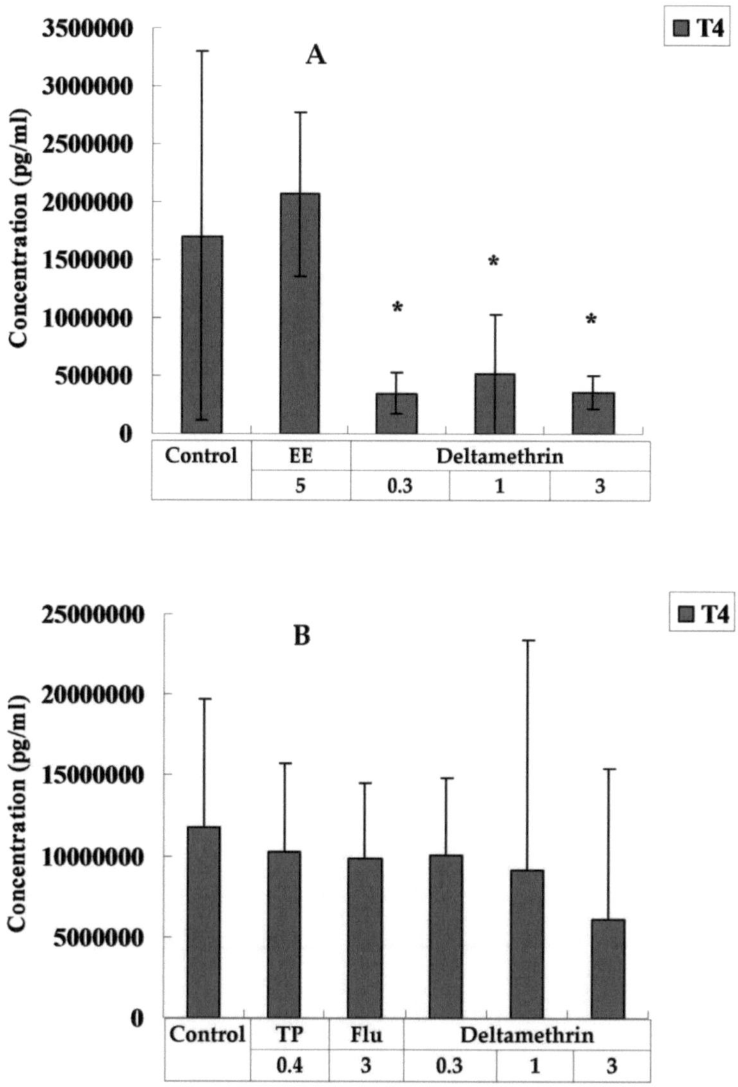

Figure 5.
Measurements of serum thyroxine (T4) treated with control, 17α-ethinyl estradiol 5 mg/kg/day (EE5) testosterone propionate 0.4 mg/kg/day (TP 0.4), flutamide 3 mg/kg/day (Flu 3), and deltamethrin 0.3, 1, and 3 mg/kg/day (Delta 0.3, Delta 1, and Delta 3) in rats. Deltamethrin significantly decreased serum T4 concentrations (A). No obvious effect was observed in male rats (B).

and reduced the mean body weight at the time of PPS to 138.9 g. However, neither deltamethrin nor flutamide affected the time or body weight at PPS, except for a reduction of body weight to 145 g induced by 3 mg/kg/day of deltamethrin (**Figure 3B**).

4.5 Effects on histology and several parameters of thyroid activity

The tissues of the thyroid glands in females and males, and the other tissues including pituitary glands (females and males), uteri, ovaries, testes, epididymides, and prostates (data not shown) of rats treated with control, EE, TP, flutamide, and deltamethrin were examined histologically. Histology of all tissues was comparable to that of the control group. No significant differences between the pituitary glands, uteri, ovaries, testes, epididymides, and prostates were detected between the controlled and treated male and female rats. Because 0.3 mg/kg/day deltamethrin

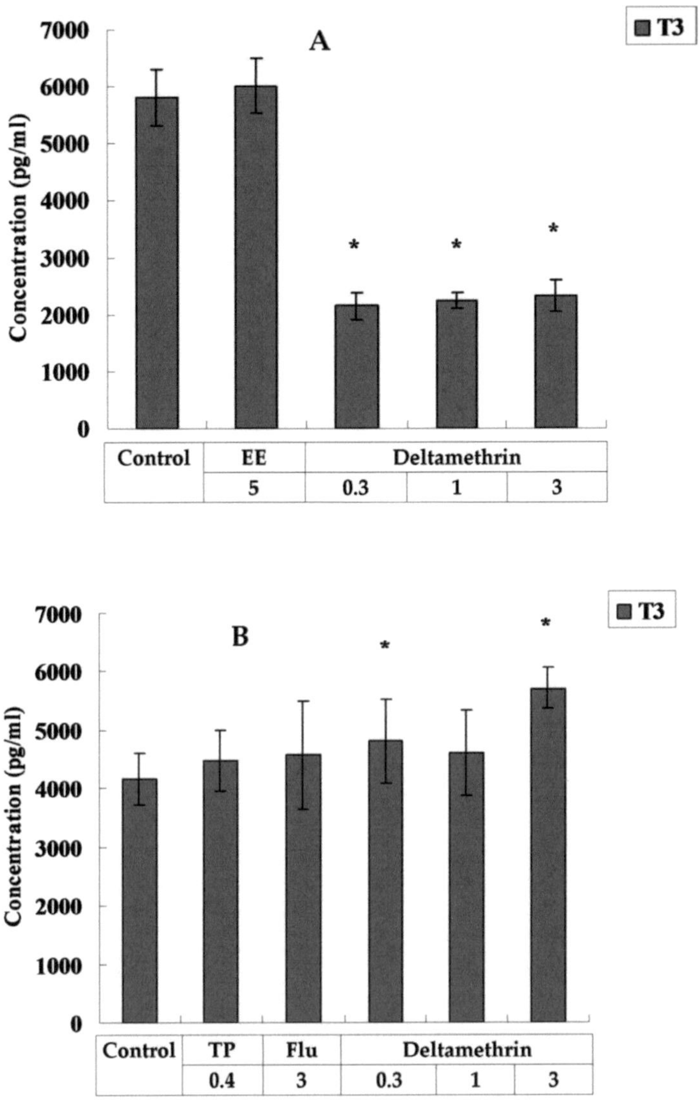

Figure 6.
Measurements of serum triiodothyronine (T3) treated with control, 17α-ethinyl estradiol 5 mg/kg/day (EE5) testosterone propionate 0.4 mg/kg/day (TP 0.4), flutamide 3 mg/kg/day (Flu 3), and deltamethrin 0.3, 1, and 3 mg/kg/day (Delta 0.3, Delta 1, and Delta 3) in rats. Deltamethrin significantly decreased T3 concentrations in female rats (A), while low and high dose significantly increased in male rats (B).

significantly reduced absolute thyroid weight (**Table 2**) and 0.3 and 1 mg/kg/day deltamethrin significantly decreased the relative thyroid weight (**Figure 2A**) in female rats, we measured the several parameters of thyroid activity. EE, TP, flutamide, and deltamethrin did not affect total area analyzed (μm^2), total colloid area (μm^2), colloid/total area (%), number of colloid, average colloid area (μm^2), average colloid diameter (μm), total epithelial area (μm^2), and epithelial/total area (%) except TP increasing average colloid area and average colloid diameter (**Table 5**).

4.6 Effects on serum hormone concentrations in female and male rats

For the female rats, EE significantly decreased serum luteinizing hormone (LH) and testosterone but increased 17ß-estradiol (E2) (**Figure 4A**) and TSH (**Figure 7A**) serum concentrations, and there is no effect on aromatase (data now

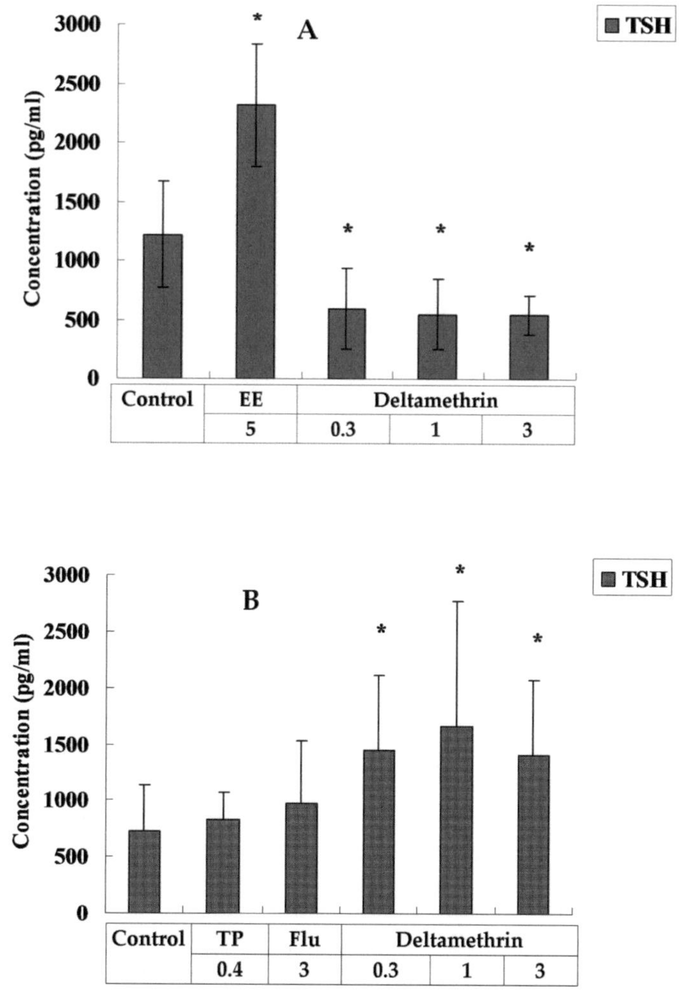

Figure 7.
Measurements of serum thyroid-stimulating hormone (TSH) treated with control, 17α-ethinyl estradiol 5 mg/kg/day (EE5) testosterone propionate 0.4 mg/kg/day (TP 0.4), flutamide 3 mg/kg/day (Flu 3), and deltamethrin 0.3, 1, and 3 mg/kg/day (Delta 0.3, Delta 1, and Delta 3) in rats. EE significantly increased TSH concentration, while deltamethrin significantly decreased it in female rats (A). In contrary to female rats, deltamethrin increased TSH concentrations in male rats (B).

shown), follicular-stimulating hormone (FSH) (data now shown), thyroxine (T4) (**Figure 5A**), and triiodothyronine (T3) (**Figure 6A**). Deltamethrin tended to decrease the serum aromatase concentration and did significantly in 1 mg/kg/day (data now shown). Deltamethrin showed no effect on serum concentrations of LH, FSH, and testosterone (data now shown). Deltamethrin significantly increased 17β-estradiol (E2) with dose-dependent manner (**Figure 4A**). Also, deltamethrin significantly decreased serum concentrations of T4 (**Figure 5A**), T3 (**Figure 6A**), and TSH (**Figure 7A**).

For the male rats, TP significantly decreased serum concentrations of LH and FSH, and there were no effect on aromatase, E2, T, T4, T3, and TSH. Flutamide significantly increased serum T, while there were no effect on aromatase (data now shown), LH (data now shown), FSH (data now shown), E2 (**Figure 4B**), T4 (**Figure 5B**), T3 (**Figure 6B**), and TSH (**Figure 7B**).

For the female rats, EE significantly increased 89% of TSH. However, deltamethrin significantly decreased 60–64% of T3, 70–80% of T4, and 51–55% of TSH concentrations. By contrast, for the male rats, 0.3 and 3 mg/kg/day of deltamethrin significantly increased 14 and 36% of T3 concentrations, and 0.3, 1, and 3 mg/kg/day deltamethrin significantly increased 100, 130, and 96% of TSH concentrations (**Table 3**).

5. Discussion

This study investigated whether deltamethrin alters pubertal development and thyroid function on the basis of previous reports regarding testicular and epididymal toxicity, neurotoxicity in juvenile/peripubertal rats, and TR antagonism in Tox21 HTS assays. Furthermore, the study was aimed at verifying whether Tox21 reporter activity data can predict the endocrine-disrupting activity of deltamethrin. Deltamethrin was observed to delay age and increase body weight at VO, accompanied with decreased T3, T4, and TSH concentrations in female rats. Based on the reductions of T3, T4, and TSH concentrations, delay in VO age, and induction of an irregular estrous cycle, we propose that deltamethrin disrupts the HPT and hypothalamic-pituitary-ovarian (HPO) axes in female rats. By contrast, deltamethrin failed to delay the age of PPS and increased T3 and TSH concentrations in the male rats. Because deltamethrin reduced T3, T4, and TSH levels in a sex-dependent manner and correlated with disturbances in pubertal development, the delay in female pubertal development might be a consequence of thyroid disruption.

The HPO axis has been demonstrated by Ortega et al. [43, 44]. Disruption of thyroid function with 133-iodine in adult female rats resulted in irregular cycles, atrophied and underweight ovaries, and decreased serum T3 and T4. However, T3 replacement restored normal cycles and ovary weights [43]. Similarly, T4 replacement restored estrous cycles and pubertal patterns of gonadotropin secretion in hypothyroid female rats [44]. Jiang et al. [45] also reported that T4 treatment improved follicular development rather than gonadotropin secretion in infertile immature hypothyroid rdw rats. By contrast, Tamura [46] reported that hypothyroidism increases ovarian hormonal secretion and folliculogenesis during equine chorionic gonadotropin-induced follicle development in immature female rats. Thus, the involvement of the HPG ovary in hypothyroidism-induced disruption of female puberty development is still unclear. In the present study, the FSH and LH levels of deltamethrin did not change (data not shown), suggesting that the HPG ovary might not be involved in the mechanism for the delay of female puberty by deltamethrin.

The results of the present study show that deltamethrin decreased concentrations of T3, T4, and TSH in female rat serums. Because the morphology of the thyroid glands was normal after deltamethrin treatment, it is unlikely that deltamethrin disturbed the biosynthesis function of TH in the thyroid glands. Given that TSH positively regulates the biosynthesis of TH, the decreases in T3 and T4 levels might be consequences of the decrease in TSH by deltamethrin. TSH is released from the anterior pituitary, which also releases LH and FSH. Because LH and FSH levels were not affected by deltamethrin, it is likely that the anterior pituitary function remained normal after deltamethrin treatment. Therefore, it is plausible that deltamethrin disturbed the regulatory mechanism for TSH synthesis or release through the anterior pituitary.

TSH is produced in pituitary thyrotrophs. It activates thyroid follicular cells and promotes thyroid cell proliferation and TH synthesis [47, 48]. TSH synthesis is largely dependent on serum TH levels. Patients with primary hyperthyroidism or primary hypothyroidism consistently demonstrate suppressed or increased serum TSH levels, respectively [49]. On the basis of the results of the present study, we infer that deltamethrin might damage TSH production or release, subsequently resulting in reductions of T3 and T4 in female rats. Furthermore, the reduction in TSH level caused by deltamethrin was sex-dependent. A possible explanation for the difference might be responsiveness to the thyrotropin-releasing hormone. The presence of a sex difference in HPT function was suggested by McClain et al. [50]. Phenobarbital increased TSH secretion as a compensatory response to the increased T4 metabolism and excretion. Higher TSH responsiveness to TRH has been observed in male rats but not in female rats, and this difference was attributed to testosterone [51]. Therefore, a possible explanation for the difference in responses to deltamethrin between male and female rats might be that male rats are more susceptible to deltamethrin than female rats are in terms of TSH response.

In contrast to the negative regulation of TSH production by THs, TSH production is positively regulated by TRH. Mice devoid of the TRH gene were shown to exhibit hypothyroidism accompanied by low circulating TSH levels and reduced numbers of TSH immunopositive cells in their pituitary glands [52]. In TRH and TR β-subunit double knockout mice, basal serum TSH levels were shown to be low and hypothyroidism failed to increase serum TSH concentrations [53]. These studies have demonstrated the pivotal role of TRH in the regulation of TSH production. The reduction of TSH in female rats might be regulated by TRH.

TSH secretion is increased by hypothyroidism [49]. In the present study, because deltamethrin increased the TSH levels in the male rats, it is possible that deltamethrin moderately reduced TH levels, which were overcome by the normal TSH regulatory system in the male rats. However, the reduction in TH levels could not activate the positive regulatory mechanism for TSH secretion in the female rats, and TH levels remained low. These results are strongly correlated with sex-dependent delay in pubertal development. A more detailed study must be conducted to elucidate the mechanisms.

Acknowledgements

We thank Sinon Co., Taichung, Taiwan, ROC, for providing deltamethrin for this study. The study was supported partly by the Bureau of Animal Plant Health Inspection and Quarantine, Council of Agriculture, Executive Yuan, ROC (104AS-10.8.1-BQ-B1), and partly by National Health Research Institutes, Zhunan, Miaoli County 35053, ROC (NHRI-105A1-PDCO-3416161).

Conflicts of interest

The authors declare no conflicts of interest.

Author details

Shui-Yuan Lu[1*], Pinpin Lin[2], Wei-Ren Tsai[1] and Chen-Yi Weng[2]

1 Applied Toxicology Division, Taiwan Agricultural Chemicals and Toxic Substances Research Institute (TACTRI), Council of Agriculture, Executive Yuan, Taichung, Taiwan, ROC

2 National Institute of Environmental Health Sciences, National Health Research Institutes (NHRI), Miaoli County, Taiwan, ROC

*Address all correspondence to: lusueyen@tactri.gov.tw

References

[1] Carson R. Silent Spring. New York: Houghton Mifflin; 1962

[2] Colborn T, vom Saal FS, Soto AM. Developmental effects of endocrine-disrupting chemicals in wildlife and humans. Environmental Health Perspectives. 1993;**101**:378-384

[3] Newbold R. Cellular and molecular effects of developmental exposure to diethylstilbestrol: Implications for other environmental estrogens. Environmental Health Perspectives. 1995;**103**(Suppl 7):83-87

[4] Ankley GT, Johnson RD, Toth G, Folman LC, Detenbeck NE, Bradbury SP. Development of a research strategy for assessing the ecological risk of endocrine disruptors. Toxicolology. 1997;**1**:71-106

[5] Kavlock RJ, Daston GP, DeRosa C, Fenner-Crisp P, Gray LE, Kaattari S, et al. Research needs for the risk assessment of health and environmental effects of endocrine disruptors: A report of the U.S. EPA-sponsored workshop. Environmental Health Perspectives. 1996;**104**(Suppl 4):715-740

[6] Endocrine Disrupter Screening and Testing Advisory Committee (EDSTAC). Endocrine Disrupter Screening and Testing Advisory Committee Final Report; 1998. Available from: http://www.epa.gov/scipoly/oscpendo/history/finalrpt.htm

[7] EPA. Pubertal Development and Thyroid Function in Intact Juvenile/Peripubertal Female Rats. Endocrine Disruptor Screening Program Test Guidelines, OPPTS 890.1450; 2009

[8] EPA. Pubertal Development and Thyroid Function in Intact Juvenile/Peripubertal Male Rats. Endocrine Disruptor Screening Program Test Guidelines, OPPTS 890.1500; 2009

[9] Brown DD, Cai LQ. Amphibian metamorphosis. Developmental Biology. 2007;**306**:20-33

[10] Carr JA, Patino R. The hypothalamus-pituitary-thyroid axis in teleosts and amphibians: Endocrine disruption and its consequences to natural populations. General and Comparative Endocrinology. 2011;**170**:299-312

[11] Wagner MS, Wajner SM, Maia AL. The role of thyroid hormone in testicular development and function. Journal of Endocrinology. 2008;**199**:351-365

[12] Wagner MS, Wajner SM, Maia AL. Is there a role for thyroid hormone on spermatogenesis? Microscopy Research and Technique. 2009;**72**:796-808

[13] Millar RP, Lu ZL, Pawson AJ, Flanagan CA, Morgan K, Maudsley SR. Gonadotropin-releasing hormone receptors. Endocrine Reviews. 2004;**25**:235-275

[14] Peper JS, Brouwer RM, van Leeuwen M, Schnack HG, Boomsma DI, Kahn RS, et al. HPG-axis hormones during puberty: A study on the association with hypothalamic and pituitary volumes. Psychoneuroendocrinology. 2010;**35**:133-140

[15] U.S. Environmental Protection Agency (EPA). Special Report on Environmental Endocrine Disruption: An Effect Assessment and Analysis. EPA/630/R-96/012. Washington, DC; 1997

[16] Andersen HR, Vinggaard AM, Rasmussen TH, Gjermandsen IM, Bonefeld-Jørgensen EC. Effects of currently used pesticides in assays for estrogenicity, androgenicity, and aromatase activity in vitro. Toxicology and Applied Pharmacology. 2002;**179**:1-12

[17] Abdallah FB, Hamden K, Galeraud-Denis I, Feki AE, Keskes-Ammar L. An in vitro study on reproductive toxicology of deltamethrin on rat spermatozoa. Andrologia. 2010;**42**:254-259

[18] Abdallah FB, Slima AB, Dammak I, Keskes-Ammar L, Mallek Z. Comparative effects of dimethoate and deltamethrin on reproductive system in male mice. Andrologia. 2010;**42**: 182-186

[19] Issam C, Samir H, Zohra H, Monia Z, Hassen BC. Toxic responses to deltamethrin (DM) low doses on gonads, sex hormones and lipoperoxidation in male rats following subcutaneous treatments. The Journal of Toxicological Sciences. 2009;**34**:663-670

[20] Oda SS, El-Maddawy ZK. Protective effect of vitamin E and selenium combination on deltamethrin-induced reproductive toxicity in male rats. Experimental and Toxicologic Pathology. 2012;**64**:813-819

[21] Ben Slima A, Ben Abdallah F, Keskes-Ammar L, Mallek Z, El Feki A, Gdoura R. Embryonic exposure to dimethoate and/or deltamethrin impairs sexual development and programs reproductive success in adult male offspring mice. Andrologia. 2012;**44**:661-666

[22] Kilian E, Delport R, Bornman MS, de Jager C. Simultaneous exposure to low concentrations of dichlorodiphenyltrichloroethane, deltamethrin, nonylphenol and phytoestrogens has negative effects on the reproductive paramethers in male Sprague-Dawley rats. Andrologia. 2007;**39**:128-135

[23] El-Gohary M, Awara WM, Nassar S, Hawas S. Deltamethrin-induced testicular apoptosis in rats: The protective effect of nitric oxide synthase inhibitor. Toxicology. 1999;**132**:1-8

[24] Dayal M, Parmar D, Dhawan A, Ali M, Dwivedi UN, Seth PK. Effect of pretreatment of cytochrome P450 (P450) modifiers on neurobehavioral toxicity induced by deltamethrin. Food and Chemical Toxicology. 2003;**41**:431-437

[25] Johri A, Dhawan A, Singh RL, Parmar D. Effect of prenatal exposure of deltamethrin on the ontogeny of xenobiotic metabolizing cytochrome P450s in the brain and liver of offsprings. Toxicology and Applied Pharmacology. 2006;**214**:279-289

[26] Yadav S, Johri A, Dhawan A, Seth PK, Parmar D. Regional specificity in deltamethrin induced cytochrome P450 expression in rat brain. Toxicology and Applied Pharmacology. 2006;**217**:15-24

[27] Magby JP, Richardson JR. Developmental pyrethroid exposure causes long-term decreases of neuronal sodium channel expression. Neurotoxicol. 2017;**60**:274-279

[28] DeMicco A, Cooper KR, Richardson JR, White LA. Developmental neurotoxicity of pyrethroid insecticides in zebrafish embryos. Toxicological Sciences. 2010;**113**:177-186

[29] Patro N, Shrivastava M, Tripathi S, Patro IK. S100β upregulation: A possible mechanism of deltamethrin toxicity and motor coordination deficits. Neurotoxicology and Teratology. 2009;**31**:169-176

[30] Lazarini CA, Florio JC, Lemonica IP, Bernardi MM. Effects of prenatal exposure to deltamethrin on forced swimming behavior, motor activity, and striatal dopamine levels in male and female rats. Neurotoxicology and Teratology. 2001;**23**:665-673

[31] Hossain MM, DiCicco-Bloom E, Richardson JR. Hippocampal ER stress and learning deficits following repeated

pyrethroid exposure. Toxicological Sciences. 2015;**143**:220-228

[32] Harrill JA, Li Z, Wright FA, Radio NM, Mundy WR, Tornero-Velez R, et al. Transcriptional response of rat frontal cortex following acute in vivo exposure to the pyrethroid insecticides permethrin and deltamethrin. BMC Genomics. 2008;**9**:546-569

[33] Armstrong LE, Driscoll MV, More VR, Donepudi AC, Xu J, Baker A, et al. Effects of developmental deltamethrin exposure on white adipose tissue gene expression. Journal of Biochemical and Molecular Toxicology. 2013;**27**:165-171

[34] Richardson JR, Taylor MM, Shalat SL, Guillot TS III, Caudle WM, Hossain MM, et al. Developmental pesticide exposure reproduces features of attention deficit hyperactivity disorder. The FASEB Journal. 2015;**29**:1960-1972

[35] Du G, Shen O, Sun H, Fei J, Lu C, Song L, et al. Assessing hormone receptor activities of pyrethroid insecticides and their metabolites in reporter gene assays. Toxicological Sciences. 2010;**116**:58-66

[36] Wang S, Shi N, Ji Z, Pinna G. Effects of pyrethroids on the concentrations of thyroid hormones in the rat serum and brain. Zhonghua Lao Dong Wei Sheng Zhi Ye Bing Za Zhi. 2002;**20**:173-176

[37] Sekeroglu V, Sekeroglu ZA, Demirhan E. Effects of commercial formulations of deltamethrin and/or thiacloprid on thyroid hormone levels in rat serum. Toxicology and Industrial Health. 2014;**30**:40-46

[38] Howdeshell KL. A model of the development of the brain as a construct of the thyroid system. Environmental Health Perspectives. 2002;**110**(Suppl 3): 337-348

[39] Merrick BA, Paules RS, Tice RR. Intersection of toxicogenomics and high throughput screening in the Tox21 program: An NIEHS perspective. International Journal of Biotechnology. 2015;**14**:7-27

[40] Everett JW. Neurobiology of Reproduction in the Female Rat: A Fifty-Year Perspective. New York: Spring-Velag; 1989

[41] Korenbrot CC, Huhtaniemi IT, Weiner RI. Preputial separation as an external sign of pubertal development in the male rat. Biology of Reproduction. 1977;**17**:298-303

[42] Capen CC, Martin SL. The effects of xenobiotics on the structure and function of thyroid follicular and C-cells. Toxicologic Pathology. 1989;**17**:266-293

[43] Ortega E, Rodriguez E, Ruiz E, Osorio C. Activity of the hypothalamo-pituitary ovarian axis in hypothyroid rats with or without triiodothyronine replacement. Life Sciences. 1990;**46**:391-395

[44] Ortega E, Osorio A, Ruiz E. Inhibition of 5'DI and 5'DII L-tiroxine (T4) monodeiodinases: Effect on the hypothalamo-pituitary ovarian axis in adult hypothyroid rats treated with T4. Biochemistry and Molecular Biology International. 1996;**39**:853-860

[45] Jiang JY, Umezu M, Sato E. Improvement of follicular development rather than gonadotrophin secretion by thyroxine treatment in infertile immature hypothyroid *rdw* rats. Journal of Reproduction and Infertility. 2000;**119**:193-199

[46] Tamura K, Hatsuta M, Watanabe G, Taya K, Kogo H. Inhibitory regulation of inhibin gene expression by thyroid hormone during ovarian development in immature rats. Biochemical and Biophysical Research Communications. 1998;**242**:102-108

[47] Magner JA. Thyroid-stimulating hormone: Biosynthesis, cell biology, and bioactivity. Endocrine Reviews. 1990;**11**:354-385

[48] Tang KT, Braverman LE, DeVito WJ. Tumor necrosis factor-alpha and interferon-gamma modulate gene expression of type I 5′-deiodinase, thyroid peroxidase, and thyroglobulin in FRTL-5 rat thyroid cells. Endocrinology. 1995;**136**:881-888

[49] Ladenson PW, Singer PA, Ain KB, Bagchi N, Bigos ST, Levy EG, et al. American Thyroid Association guidelines for detection of thyroid dysfunction. Archives of Internal Medicine. 2000;**160**:1573-1575

[50] McClain RM, Posch RC, Bosakowski T, Armstrong JM. Studies on the mode of action for thyroid gland tumor promotion in rats by phenobarbital. Toxicology and Applied Pharmacology. 1988;**94**:254-265

[51] Christianson D, Roti E, Vagenakis AG, Braverman LE. The sex related difference in serum thyrotropin concentration is androgen mediated. Endocrinology. 1981;**108**:529-535

[52] Yamada M, Saga Y, Shibusawa N, Hirato J, Murakami M, Iwasaki T, et al. Tertiary hypothyroidism and hyperglycemia in mice with targeted disruption of the thyrotropin-releasing hormone gene. Proceedings of the National Academy of Sciences. 1997;**94**:10862-10867

[53] Nikrodhanond AA, Ortiga-Carvalho TM, Shibusawa N, Hashimoto K, Liao XH, Refetoff S, et al. Dominant role of thyrotropin-releasing hormone in the hypothalamic-pituitary-thyroid axis. Journal of Biological Chemistry. 2006;**281**:5000-5007

Chapter 4

A Review on the Influence of Climate Change on Sheep Reproduction

Gregory Sawyer and Edward Jitik Narayan

Abstract

Increasing food and natural fibre production ensure food security for nearly 10 billion people, the projected global population in 2050, without causing further environmental damage can be achieved by transforming systems and adopting sustainable agriculture practices within a changing climate. Globally, climate change effects are having both direct and indirect effects on agricultural productivity including changing rainfall patterns, drought, flooding and the geographical redistribution of pests and diseases. Climate change induced heat stress is thus one of the complex factors making sheep management and husbandry challenging in many geographical locations in the world. Within the sheep industry, reproductive wastage (RW) is a major challenge throughout the varying breeding landscapes. Reproductive wastage is defined as the early losses of embryos undergoing natural and/or artificial breeding programs. Our previous research showed that heat stress (THI > 75) and elevated glucocorticoid levels (indexed using faecal glucocorticoid metabolites) are linked to embryo loss in Merino ewes. This mini review discusses how extreme variation in climate such as heat stress affects the maternal reproductive performance in the Merino sheep and the impacts on the wool industry. We provide recommendations to sheep producers for monitoring and managing the effects of heat stress on-farm.

Keywords: reproductive wastage, stress, merino sheep, climate change, resilience, production

1. Introduction

1.1 Interaction between climate, human population and sheep reproduction

As the world's global climate is changing, the United Nations is projecting a global population of nearly 10 billion people by 2050 [1]. It is thus the graziers, farmers and pastoralists who are charged with feeding this population growth, like they have always done since the beginning of time. However, within this changing global climate, domestic animal farmers (sheep, cattle, goats and pigs) will be required to engage with not only the buyers of their products (to show sustainable practices) but also with their environment better by transforming on farm systems through adoption of better sustainable agriculture practices within this changing climate [1].

Globally, climate change has both direct and indirect effects on agricultural productivity including changing rainfall patterns, drought, flooding and the geographical redistribution of pests and diseases [1]. Climate is one of the three key influences that affect the welfare (health and well-being) of livestock with the others being, nutrition management, external and internal diseases. Synergy among these three key components influences the physiological and phenotypic/behavioural responses of livestock and ultimate productivity.

Recent developments in the field of animal welfare such as non-invasive technology can assess animal emotion and pain and have led to wider interests from researchers and advocate for animal welfare directed research in production animal systems [3], especially in Australia, as a vast and dynamic country which regularly experiences extreme climatic conditions [2].

Livestock animals pioneered into Australia are mostly of the European breed, so they have to cope with the daily challenges presented by the Australian climate, ranging from sub-freezing winters to moderately hot summers. Advancements in the dynamics of Australian agriculture over the past half-century have been channelled mainly through human innovations in machinery, nutrition and animal genetics. These advancements are supplemented with better equipped personalised technologies to predict climatic events [4] including above and below above average rainfall or radiant heat loads. However, within Australia, since 1910 the average maximum day time temperature has increased by 0.7°C and a night time temperature increase of 1.1°C, with much of this change occurring since the industrial revolution in the 1950s.

Since the 1940s, small scale research shows that the reproductive potential of Merino ewes may be negatively influenced by one or a combination of environmental factors. In the 1960s and 1970s, key research into heat stress and its influence in RW provided evidence that environmental stress can heavily influence reproductive success in the Merino sheep [5–8]. Previous research into fertility and reproductive ability in mammals also demonstrated, through a wide variety of trials and scientific reviews, the physiological responses associated with the perception or recognition of internal or external stressors [9, 10]. Most recently, Narayan et al. [11] determined that summer heat wave can impact the management outcomes of commercial livestock reproduction programs involved in artificial insemination (AI) and embryo transfer (ET) through the generation of physiological stress and early loss of embryos in 'hot ewes' [11]. New research into how climatic induced heat stress represents a physiological challenge to normal expression of life-history traits such as growth, development, behaviour and reproduction in domesticated farm animals is gaining interest throughout the agricultural sector worldwide. In domestic food animals (e.g., Merino ewe and Angus cow), reproductive ability is the most economically important trait that may be compromised by changing environments and subsequent stress [12].

1.2 Current demographics in Australia

Australia is the world's largest apparel wool growing country (80%), with 100% of all wool produced exported throughout the world. In 2007, the Australian Bureau of Statistics (ABS) reported the total Australian flock numbers of 85.7 million head [13]. The number of breeding ewes (of all breeds) equated to 46.4 million head of the total sheep population in 2007 [14]. The 2017 joint Meat and Livestock Australia (MLA) and Australian Wool Innovation (AWI) quartile report on wool and sheep meat provided sheep numbers, both Merino and other breeds, at vastly reduced levels not seen for generations [16]. According to the ABS (**Table 1**), as of the 30th June 2017 the total Australian flock numbers had reduced to 72.15 million head [17]. The breeding ewe population as of the 30th of June 2017 within Australia was 39.89 million breeding ewes which represent a reduction of 6.51 million breeding ewes aged 1 year and older [19].

	Number of head
Breeding ewes 1 year and older [including merinos and all other breeds]	39,897,000
Lambs under 1 year old	22,857,000
All other sheep and lambs	9,371,000
Total sheep in Australia of all breeds and all ages	72,125,000

Source: Australian Bureau of Statistics 2016–2017 End of Financial Year Livestock Numbers (Australian Bureau of Statistics, 2018 [16]).

Table 1.
Australian total sheep population (number of head): as of 30th June 2017.

In 2011, ABS reported a total of 40,000 sheep businesses in Australia only 9814 of which are Merino-based operations [13]. This number had reduced to 31,136 in the ABS 2015–2016 censuses [14].

1.2.1 Wool volume

According to AWI, the volume of all wool tested through the Australian Wool Testing Authority (AWTA) Ltd. has been relatively stable over the past six financial years 2009/2010–2016/2017. During that period the tested volume has been revolving around 360 million kg greasy plus or minus 5% [15].

1.2.2 Sheepmeat volume

Australia is the world's largest exporter of sheepmeat, and the world's second largest producer of lamb and mutton [17]. In 2014–2015, the sheepmeat industry accounted for 32% of all farms in Australia with agricultural activity [14]. The off-farm meat value (domestic expenditure plus export value) of the Australian sheepmeat industry was approximately AUD[1] $4.83 billion in 2015–2016—up 2% on the 2014–2015 periods (MLA estimate).

1.2.3 Climatic and sheep number changes

In the period 1880–2012, the surface global warming was 0.85°C and 2015 was the warmest in the instrumental record [18]. Heatwaves in 2013 (Australia's hottest year), 2014 and 2015 had substantial impacts on infrastructure, health, electricity supply, transport and agriculture [18]. When we compare this climate change increase in heating of the Australian land and sea environments between 2012 and 2016, 32 of the 39 geographical areas, as determined by Meat and Livestock Australia, had decreases in sheep populations up to 41% of the 2011 total. Appendix 1 provides information on sheep population change between 2012–2013 and 2015–2016 financial years as provided by Meat and Livestock Australia [19].

2. Climate change

Climate change is defined as the long-term misbalance of customary weather conditions such as temperature, wind and rainfall characteristics of a specific

[1] AUD-Australian Dollar Value

region and it is likely to be one of the main challenges that mankind faces during the present century [20]. Climatic change impacts on agriculture and livestock are being witnessed all around the world [21, 24, 25]. The United Nations Food and Agriculture Organisation [59] in 2008 recognised that throughout the world, there is increasing general agreement that the direct effects of climate change will be of a similar nature in both low and high-external input livestock production systems.

The Earth's climate is predicted to continually change at rates unprecedented in recent human history [20, 22]. Current climate models indicate a 0.28°C temperature increase per decade for the next two decades and predict the increase in global average surface temperature by 2100 may be between 1.88 and 4.08°C [20, 22]. According to NASA [23], the global average surface temperature increased from 0.6 to 0.9°C between 1906 and 2005, and the *rate* of temperature increase has nearly doubled in the last 50 years. The Earth's climate has warmed dramatically in the last century, with the 1990s and 2000s being the warmest on instrumental record [20, 22]. A selection of global climate models projects the average Australian temperature relative to 1990 to increase by 0.1–1.3°C by 2020, 0.3–3.4°C by 2050 and up to 6.7°C by 2080 [26].

3. Climate change and thermal stress

Within an animal breeding environment, ambient temperature is a most important variable as its effect is aggravated in the presence of high humidity [27]. Concerningly, as temperature and humidity levels increase over much of the continent [28] amplified thermal stress on animals is expected. Thermal (heat) stress is defined as any combination of environmental parameters producing conditions that are higher than the temperature range of the animal's thermoneutral zone (TNZ) [30]. Thermal stress can adversely affect a range of reproduction indices, including a suppressive effect on reproductive hormones [31].

Pregnant and lactating ruminants are more susceptible to heat stress than non-pregnant and non-lactating individuals [32, 33, 53]. As the animal is affected by heat stress, via HPA activation the animal reduces its reproduction role within both the male (sperm mobility, sperm abnormalities) and in the female (through reduced oestrous activity, embryonic mortality) [33]. Physiologically, the metabolic changes within the animal due to the influence of heat stress can be assessed in a sheep through non-invasive assessment methods. Chronic stress can be measured in raw wool samples as well as progesterone to determine pregnancy in stressed and non-stressed sheep [29]. Those ewes which are affected by heat stress and heat shock acutely can have through non-invasive methods have faecal matter tested for stress [29].

In cattle, Dash [34] showed a negative correlation between reproduction traits, temperature humidity index (THI) with animals experiencing adverse effects of heat stress when the THI crosses a threshold level greater than 75.

Due to the size of Australia and the location of the Australian sheep breeding areas (tablelands, grasslands, rangelands, arid) various physical environmental stressors (PES) are dynamic and can be localised or decentralised within the greater region. PES include: high ambient temperature, high direct and indirect solar radiation, wind speed, and relative humidity. Among the physical environmental stressors, ambient temperature is ecologically the most important [47]. PES can cause the effective temperature of the environment to often exceed the TNZ of the animals [43], leading to heat stress [44–46].

In sheep, Narayan et al. [11] showed that heat stress reduces embryo production during AI/ET because the physiological and cellular aspects of reproductive function and early embryo development are disrupted. Thus, climatic change induced heat stress can diminish reproductive capacity in the Merino ewe due to an increase in body temperature as it is exposed to elevated ambient temperature, and by the physiological adaptations of cells coping with thermal stress [35, 36].

In Merino sheep, elevated maternal cortisol levels caused by thermal stress can lead to a programming of the hypothalamic-pituitary-adrenal (HPA) axis. It has emerged that this HPA axis programming is a possible key mechanism [37, 38] resulting in the foetal adaptation to its environment; the placenta acts as a connection between the mother and the developing foetus and stress activates maternal HPA axis functioning and triggers glucocorticoid (GC) secretion that reaches the foetus by transplacental passage [39]. Glover's [39] research confers that behaviours and health outcomes in an offspring may result from long-lasting endocrine changes between the maternal-foetal nexus guided by complex networks of hormones (e.g., glucocorticoids, insulin-like growth factors-IGFs and hormones expressed along the brain-gut axis) [39]. With sheep breeding enterprises impact of climate change that causes GC secretion may induce epigenetic changes within individual animals among larger sheep populations—the effect of which will have long lasting changes to the DNA of future disease resistance, reproduction capacity and nutritional conversions in the future off spring(s) [89].

Heat stress is qualified as cytotoxic, as it alters biological molecules, disturbs cell functions, modulates metabolic reactions, induces oxidative cell damage and activates both apoptosis and necrosis pathways [33, 40]. Epigenetic modifications can also occur in the offspring of pregnant ewes in response to external or internal environmental factors (i.e., heat stress and water stress). Heat stress is thus one of the complex factors making sheep management and husbandry challenging in many geographical locations in the world [42, 98].

3.1 Climate change and sheep welfare

Climatic change that causes chronic heat stress is considered the most important external factor drastically affecting long term small ruminant (sheep) reproduction globally [21, 51, 52]. Since domestication, sheep have established a wide geographical range due to their adaptability to nutrient-rich and nutrient-poor diets, along with tolerance to extreme climatic conditions [41].

Australian vast land mass and varying weather and changing climatic challenges are dominant features. Thus, Australian sheep of all breeds are exposed to not only a progressively warming climate, but, superimposed on that, to more frequent and extreme heat waves and droughts [48]. As a result, a warming climate that accompanies both a nutrition and water shortage is likely to present a severe challenge to a sheep homeostasis during periods of prolonged droughts.

As the environment imposes a heat load on sheep, which it will do increasingly as air temperatures rise, the only way for sheep to lose that heat and their metabolic heat is through evaporative cooling [49]. This mechanism is particularly important for sheep exposed to solar radiation. The cooling mechanism of thermoregulation in sheep will be challenged as they are small ruminants and homeotherms, so they must regulate their body temperature within a narrow range (38.5–39.5°C) to remain healthy and productive.

Thermoregulation is crucial to mammalian climate change resilience. Those sheep that are not suited or acclimatised via thermoregulation to thermal stress caused by heating of environmental conditions can result in significant elevation in body temperature which influences ovarian function, oestrus expression, oocyte health and embryonic development [34].

Within these challenges driven by the climatic change, sheep producers should anticipate changes in preimplantation environmental conditions (1), the uterine and placental competency (2), and adequate nutrient transport across the placenta (3), all of which are stressors that can all alter foetal development trajectories [50]. Alliston and Ulberg [54], Sawyer [7] and recently Narayan et al. [11] provided concise evidence that ewes subject to high air temperature at time of mating will have a reduced reproductive rate through embryo loss [8, 11, 54]. Thermal stress is also known to influence the superovulation response in sheep [55] and cattle [56, 57] in a multiple ovulation and embryo transfer program (MOET) [58].

Due to climate change, the frequency of catastrophic events (drought, flood, ambient temperature decrease, and increase), as well as possible disease epidemics and water scarcity, there is an increase in physiological stress, reduced productivity and genetic losses [59]. How well sheep are able to buffer the effects of climate change [48] will directly affect reproductive fitness, through the effects of heat stress on physiological tolerance, performance and reproductive capacity. Therefore, within the various Australian sheep breeding climates, the Australian Merino ewe will be affected by increased climatic stress experienced in either winter or summer, as seasonal conditions change with climate change.

3.2 Adaptation to thermal stress

Evidence suggests that differences exist between domesticated ruminant species, breed and production level that will influence heat stress susceptibility [60, 61] and subsequent heat stress adaptation. This is mainly due to species' differences in the ability to reduce metabolic and endogenous heat production and increase heat dissipation. For instance, animals adapted to hot environments have lower metabolic and water turnover rates, and a higher capacity to dissipate heat via panting and sweating [62] Among species, sheep and goats are considered less sensitive to heat stress than cattle [60, 63].

There is evidence for a temporal biphasic pattern of heat acclimation: short-term and long-term heat acclimations (STHA and LTHA, respectively) [64–66]. STHA is the phase in which changes are initiated within cellular signalling pathways [64] leading to disturbances in cellular homeostasis that begins to reprogram cells to survive the deleterious effects of heat stress [66]. In rodents, the full expression of STHA is attained when the plasmatic thyroid hormones (T3 and T4) levels exceeds 30–40% [66].

In ruminants, the STHA is characterised by responses initiated to compensate for the increased heat stress before permanent acclimation can be obtained. Increased heat dissipation (primarily through evaporative heat loss), reduces feed intake. Milk yield, increased water intake and tender wool in woollen sheep breeds are examples of the STHA response [52]. Within various long-term and short-term climate change projections, research continually show that biophysical events directly impact on livestock affecting nutrition requirements and reproductive success [20].

Wool is a natural indicator of short-term stress exposure within the sheep's natural environment. Wool fibres reduce in microns at the point of stress caused by individual events or through a combination of factors (nutrition, disease or pregnancy) (**Figure 1**). As the animal grows the wool throughout the wool growing period (normally 12 months), visual assessment along, within wool testing laboratory that can determine key stress periods in animals that have experienced STHA. However, LTHA exposure to nutritional stress along the full wool growth period will not see

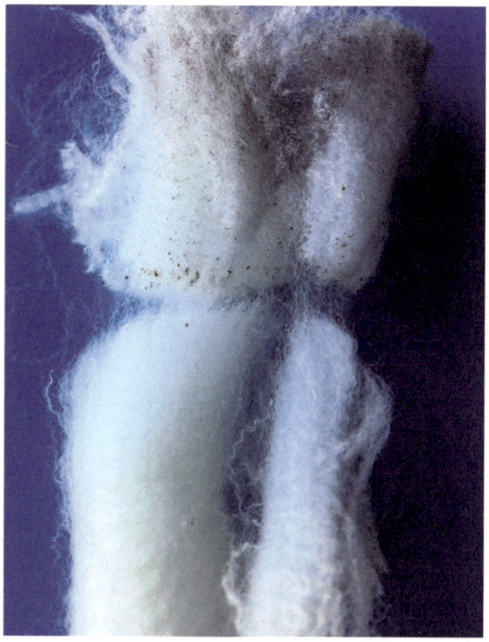

Figure 1.
An example of tender fleece and the occurrence of a fleece break. Source: Approval from Ooranook pastoral company private photo collection 2018.

the wool break as the animal is on a constant plane of nutrition. The fibre may still break however if the animal develops STHA disease or pregnancy stress while being nutritionally challenged.

When the initial acclimation phase is complete, and the heat-acclimated phenotype is expressed, LTHA occurs [47, 66]. LTHA is characterised by a reprogrammed gene expression and cellular response resulting in enhanced efficiency of signalling pathways and metabolic processes [47], and this, in large part, may be mediated by heat shock proteins (HSP) [67].

The phase of acclimation is also characterised by endocrine changes presumably with the goal of decreasing metabolic heat production and increasing heat dissipation. An example of LTHA is an ewe's body temperature that is chronically (for 40–45 days) heat-stressed (THI = 82), presenting similar results as those reported for heifers [20, 68] and cows [20, 68] In cattle, heat stress has also been associated with impaired embryo development and increased embryo mortality [35, 36, 83] see **Figure 2** for ewe effect to heat stress.

Mittal and Ghosh [69] provide key research that shows animals that can maintain or adjust physiological responses within normal limits under stressful environmental conditions may be considered adapted to that environment and hence worth rearing commercially [58, 69]. This research, when used alongside current maternal nutrition research [70, 71], suggests that animals have a prenatal growth trajectory which is sensitive to both direct and indirect effects of both maternal nutrition and stressful environmental conditions at all stages between oocyte maturation and birth [71, 72].

The biological mechanism by which heat stress impacts animal production and reproduction is partly explained by reduced feed intake. However, it also includes an altered endocrine status, reduction in rumination and nutrient absorption, and increased maintenance requirements [61] resulting in a net decrease in nutrient/energy availability. Naturally, a reduction in energy intake, combined with increased energy expenditure for maintenance, lowers the energy balance, and

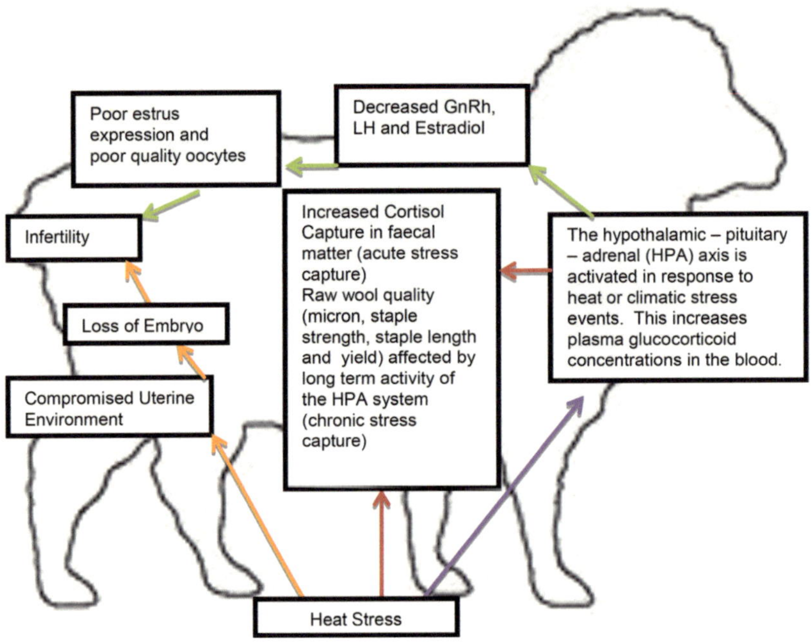

Figure 2.
Climate change induced heat stress effect on the Ovis aries: increased cortisol capture in faecal (STHA) and wool (LTHA), HPA axis activates, decreased hormones, poor estrus and lower quality oocytes, compromised uterine environment, loss of embryo leading to infertility.

partially explains why lactating cattle lose a significant amount of body weight during severe heat stress [20, 72, 73]. Reduction in energy intake coupled with increased maintenance costs during heat stress causes negative energy balance (NEBAL) in lactating cows (likely stage of lactation independent) and a bioenergetic state, similar (but not into the same extent) to the NEBAL observed in early lactation. The NEBAL associated with the early post-partum period is coupled with increased risk of metabolic disorders and health problems, decreased milk yield and reduced reproductive performance [20, 74]. Similarly, we hypothesise that many of the negative effects of heat stress on Merino production, health and reproduction indices might be mediated by NEBAL.

However, in ewes, as with cows, further research is required to know how much of the reduction in performance (yield and reproduction) can be attributed or accounted directly (hyperthermia) or indirectly (reduced feed intake) to heat stress [20]. Heat stress acclimation is accomplished by changes in homeostatic responses [47] and may include homeorhetic/teleophoretic processes involving an altered endocrine status that ultimately affects target tissue responsiveness to environmental stimuli. Initial responses are considered for homeostatic mechanisms and these include increased water intake, sweating and respiration rates, reduced heart rate and feed intake [47, 75]. Hormones are also implicated in the acclimatory response to heat stress [61] and they primarily include thyroid hormones, prolactin, GH, glucocorticoids and mineral corticoids.

Furthermore, protein synthesis as well as deoxyribonucleic acid (DNA) and ribonucleic acid (RNA) polymerisation is disrupted under heat stress. Whereas protein and RNA synthesis recover rapidly after heat exposure, DNA synthesis remains inhibited for a longer period [76, 77]. Further, heat stress is responsible of protein denaturation, and also induces their aggregation into the nuclear matrix. This aggregation increases the nuclear protein concentration [76, 77]. Therefore, many molecular functions are altered, such as DNA synthesis, replication and repair, cellular division and nuclear enzymes and DNA polymerases functions [78]. Further research is required on how heat induced stress can lead to epigenetic change in the DNA of offspring and subsequent phenotype.

Accurately identifying heat-stressed ruminants and understanding the biological mechanism(s) by which thermal stress reduces reproductive indices, milk synthesis and growth, is critical for developing novel stock management approaches (i.e., genetic, managerial and nutritional). This is particularly important for Australian Merino sheep producers, to understand as it influences production traits and reproduction capacity, especially during periods of thermal (heat) stress.

4. Reproductive wastage

Lamb marking percentages in Australia have changed little for many generations [79, 80], despite improvements in breeding, nutrition and tools for managing pregnant ewes [80, 81]. The wider influence and effects of climate change on lamb marking percentages is yet to be researched. However, climate induced heat stress during pregnancy is known to slow down foetal growth and increase foetal loss [20]. Even in favourable seasons, across a range of different sheep enterprises, lamb losses in order of 10–30% for single and twin bearing ewes, respectively, are to be expected [82]. In lead in years to the 2018 drought in New South Wales and Queensland, many regions experienced very little rain fall, cold dry winters, hot summers and vastly lowered nutritional benefit from grazing productive pastures resulting in many sheep graziers having reproductive wastage (RW) in excess of 60% in their sheep populations.

Within Australia, Merino lives and reproduces in complex macro (tropical, temperate, arid) and micro environments in which they are constantly confronted with short- and long-term environmental changes caused by a wide range of factors [27]. Embryo development within the micro-environment formed by the oviduct and uterus is influenced by the outside environment [35, 36]. If a moderate climatic change causes an increase in temperature beyond the TNZ of the maternal ewe, the cellular environment surrounding the embryo, and needed for development and growth, can be impacted. Thus, the body temperature of Merino female around the time of mating is vital for reproductive success.

Within various ruminants like sheep there are genetic differences with respect to heat stress adaptations and these may provide clues or tools to select productive and thermotolerant animals. These differences include the role of Heat Shock Proteins (HSP) in coordinating thermotolerance, the quality of the ova, the incidence of oestrus and the asynchrony between conceptus and uterus at implantation. The association between polymorphisms within the HSP genes suggests a better understanding of these relationships would help identify positive production traits and factors that impact physiological response to heat stress.

The magnitude of either one of the three key influences that affect the welfare (health and well-being) of livestock, these being climate, nutrition management and external and internal diseases, can impact oocyte quality and thereby influence fertility [84]. The quality of the oocyte is a crucial component in determining reproduction wastage. Oocyte and/or embryo quality is most affected when ewes are exposed to a hot environment during the first 3 days after artificial insemination [8]. High internal body temperature > 39.5°C leads to high cortisol (stress) levels and subsequently reduced levels of transferable eggs in AI/ET [11].

In previous research, Lindsay et al. [85] found no significant relationship between mean maximum temperature and the incidence of oestrus for Merino flocks in Western Australia [85]. However, in the same study the authors identified a negative correlation between the ambient temperature and lambing performance, but only when a higher temperature coincided with the time of mating or the few weeks thereafter. Within the South Australia environment, Kleemann and Walker [86] observed a significant decline (97–87%) in fertility as mean maximum temperatures increased <32°Cover three or more days [86]. They concluded that the reductions in lambing performance were due to increases in embryo mortality (a direct indicator of reproductive wastage). Dutt [5, 9] and Thwaites [7] in the 1960s and 1970s concluded that increasing environmental ambient temperatures within 8 days prior to conception, as well as high post-mating temperatures (within 2–3 weeks post joining), had also significantly reduced embryo survival rates. Narayan et al. [11], expanding on this earlier research, found that acute heat stress, elevated rectal temperature and elevated cortisol could adversely affect the fertility of Merino ewes.

A complication affecting the reproductive capacity in ewes is the asynchrony between conceptus and uterus at implantation [87] with as many as one-fourth of all successful fertilizations not result in a viable pregnancy, even in the absence of environmental stressors [88].

4.1 Nutritional affect

The connection between nutrition and the outcomes of reproduction in sheep extensively researched for over 50 years in Australian sheep [4–7, 18, 19, 29, 30, 45, 55, 65, 67, 77, 78, 90]. A major key determinant of the reproductive success in ewes is the relation between their live body weight (BW) and their body shape and her body condition score (BCS). Both BW and BCS (in a five-point score where 1 BCS is very low to BCS 5 is very fat: 3 BCS is ideal for joining) have a direct relationship with nutrition and water quality from pre joining, post joining and post lambing periods. If the ewe has access to continual low-quality nutrition throughout pre and post pregnancy, her reserves of body fat will be metabolised to assist with supporting herself and her unborn or recently born lamb. Previous research by Ferguson et al. [70] noted that the nutritional requirements of the ewe can be difficult to predict due to the difference in the ewe and unborn lambs′ energy requirements. Ferguson et al. [70] determined that nutritional intake capacity was influenced by the point of pregnancy and lactation and the number of lambs born and reared.

Researchers of this paper have observed hundreds of thousands of ewe(s) of various breeds within different climate zones in Australia since 1987–2019. It was noticeable that ewes with low BCS had low metabolised fat reserves, thus it appeared and could be determined that the ewe was under greater nutritional stress (especially caused through climatic events such as drought or floods). Individual ewe management is important with ewes with very low BCS (1–2.25 points) during pregnancy required to be given alternative feed to lift convertible nutrition outcomes. This is particularly important, as researchers and farmers have observed in paddock scenario's the ewe putting her survival before her embryos and aborting the unborn lamb. If the lamb is newly born (usually within 7 days), it is not uncommon for the ewe to walk away from the lamb so that she can survive. This is mostly seen in low and very low BCS ewes who have subsequent reduced nutritional energy, poor lactation and may have been affected by climatic nutritional stress (in particular drought and flood events).

As BW and BCS can significantly influence the fertility and fecundity of breeding ewes [70, 91–93], Borg et al. [94] estimated positive correlations between the number of lambs born and maternal body weight change during late gestation which could be achieved with various on farm management practices including shearing patterns and feeding regimes [94]. This seems to further support the postulation that epigenetic factors such as nutrition and climatic factors can influence the maternal environment and influence the outcome of conception with either successful breeding or embryo/lamb loss.

4.2 Heat stress and reproductive wastage

Previous research by Dutt [5, 9], Thwaites [7], Sawyer [8], Naqvi et al. [58], and Narayan et al. [11] provide evidence that ewes which are subjected to high air temperature (<32°C) at time of mating will have a reduced reproductive rate due to an increased embryonic death rate. Ewes selected on the basis of their tolerance to heat stress indicate that the group selected for lower rectal temperature had higher joining (89% vs. 63%) and lamb marking rates (82% vs. 50%) than those selected for high rectal temperature ≥ 39.9°C [95].

The inability of the animal to manage any combination of environmental conditions (i.e., air temperature, relative humidity, solar radiation) above the ewe's TNZ [41] is a prime cause of heat stress and RW. Given the rate of climate change and the near-term acceleration in the rate of temperature change within ecologically critical terrestrial climate conditions, many animals alive now will experience biologically significant climate change within their expected lifetimes [48].

While there are several possible mechanisms by which heat stress can prevent the growth of oocytes, the primary response, as determined in cattle and shown by Dash [34], is the reduction on the synthesis of preovulatory surge in the luteinizing hormone and estradiol [34]. Dash's research [34], followed by Hansen's work [35, 36], showed that due to heat stress, there was also poor follicle maturation and this leads to ovarian inactivity in cattle [34–36]. Khodaei-Motlagh [96], by determining reproductive hormones in dairy cattle in 2011, showed that heat stress delays follicle selection and reduces the degree of dominance of the dominant follicle [96]. This echoes an earlier study in 2003 that indicated heat stress may reduce summer fertility in dairy and beef cattle by causing poor estrous expression due to reduced estradiol secretion from the dominant follicle developing in a low luteinizing hormone environment [101], and that the dominant follicle is susceptible to heat stress [100]. The reason for the delay to onset of estrus could be due to a modified pulsatile release of LH and a decrease in oestrogen secretion. The normal GnRH release patterns (and subsequent frequency and amplitude of LH pulses secreted from the pituitary) are reduced by exposure to thermal stress [99]. This lack of function due to climatic pressures of heat and humidity can result in abnormal ovarian functions and hence cause a delay in the LH surge [58].

In evolutionary terms, when fertility of an individual ewe's is reduced by heat stress, the dominance of the selected follicle is reduced in consequence of a reduction of the steroidogenic capacity of theca and granulosa cells driving a fall in blood estradiol concentrations [101]. It is also widely accepted that heat stress induces a percentage of infertility in animals not suited or acclimatised internally to thermal stress. As with all homeotherms, the Merino ewe has the ability to rid itself of this sub-vital energy drain (i.e., pregnancy) due to the additional stress caused by the extreme climate which becomes a trade-off for immediate health and survival [87].

5. Final considerations

In varying sheep breeding regions, producers are likely to see a substantial increase in the frequency of heat stress days above their normal climatic conditions that may result in reduced productivity and decreased reproductive rates [102].

The ewe is the driving force of the wool and sheep meat industry, both locally and globally, as it provides both Merino and cross bred lambs and furthermore, passes valuable genetics on to the next generation [11]. In sheep reproduction and endocrinology there is now an increasingly urgent industry desire and need for further research on the physiological changes in ewes caused by climate change.

As sheep are small ruminants and homeotherms they must regulate their body temperature within a narrow range to remain healthy and productive. Heat stress is thus considered the most important factor affecting small ruminant production under changing climatic conditions [21, 51, 52]. When the physiological mechanisms in ruminants/sheep fail to alleviate the effect of heat load due to climatic changes in the environment, the body's high temperature may increase to a point at which animal well-being and reproductive capacity is compromised [5–11].

Due to the various combinations of factors such as temperature, humidity, wind and direct and indirect radiations [20] various stressors (heat cold, nutritional, disease) will be an ever-present feature of life for sheep farmers. Along with epigenetic (non-genomic) patterns resulting in altered embryo and neonate survival rates [97] the effects of climate change are one of the three key influences that affect the welfare (health and well-being) of sheep, and all livestock, with the others being nutrition management and external and internal diseases. These three key influences may cause STHA or LTHA stressors and their interaction is likely to add to and exacerbate existing pastoral gazing management challenges to sheep producers that compromise animal nutrition and health [101, 102] and subsequently reduce reproductive performance.

This review then confirms earlier research by Thwaites [7], Sawyer [8], Dutt [5, 9] and Narayan [11] that exposure of ewes to high ambient temperatures at various stages of the reproductive cycle has a detrimental effect on fertilisation rate and embryo survival. Therefore, with an increase in ambient temperatures due to climate change we hypothesis that as the climate continues to warm, the fertility of ewes will be compromised without individual management technology assessment, that is, individual health monitor located in an ear tag.

New research would provide a greater understanding of how the current sheep breed performance is challenged by the thermal environment and how on-farm practices could be improved through the application of innovative tools to assess animal welfare. Such research would help to optimise technology for making on-farm data collection (e.g., reproductive cycles) available more easily and in-real time (e.g., through applications of digital ear-tag technologies). It is acknowledged that for further growth and prosperity into the future, the sheep industry needs to proactively develop out of square thinking and innovative approaches to meet the challenge of climatic change. This would help promote positive growth into the future of the global sheep industries and wider livestock industry.

Author details

Gregory Sawyer* and Edward Jitik Narayan*
School of Science and Health, Western Sydney University, Penrith, NSW, Australia

*Address all correspondence to: 19157610@student.westernsydney.edu.au and e.narayan@westernsydney.edu.au

References

[1] United Nations Food and Agricultural Organisation. Climate Change. Food and Agriculture Organization of the United Nations; 2018. Retrieved from: http://www.fao.org/climate-change/en/

[2] Head L, Adams M, McGregor H, Toole S. Climate change and Australia. Wiley Interdisciplinary Reviews: Climate Change. 2013;**5**(2):175-197. DOI: 10.1002/wcc.255

[3] Grandin T. Improving Animal Welfare: A Practical Approach, 2nd ed.; 2015

[4] Henry B, Charmley E, Eckard R, Gaughan J, Hegarty R. Livestock production in a changing climate: Adaptation and mitigation research in Australia. Crop and Pasture Science. 2012;**63**(3):191-202. DOI: 10.1071/cp11169

[5] Dutt B, Mills C. Reproductive failure in rats due to copper deficiency. Journal of Comparative Pathology and Therapeutics. 1960;**70**:120-125. DOI: 10.1016/s0368-1742(60)80010-0

[6] Smith I. Reproductive wastage in Merino sheep in semi-arid tropical Queensland: Observations on flock mated during the spring and summer. Australian Journal of Experimental Agriculture. 1965;**5**(17):110-114. DOI: 10.1071/ea9650110

[7] Thwaites C. Short term heat stress and embryo mortality in the ewe. Australian Journal of Experimental Agriculture. 1971;**11**(50):265-267. DOI: 10.1071/ea9710265

[8] Sawyer G. The influence of radiant heat load on reproduction in the Merino ewe. II. The relative effects of heating before and after insemination. Australian Journal of Agricultural Research. 1979;**30**(6):1143-1149. DOI: 10.1071/ar9791143

[9] Dutt R. Critical period for early embryo mortality in ewes exposed to high ambient temperature. Journal of Animal Science. 1963;**22**(3):713-719. DOI: 10.2527/jas1963.223713x

[10] Nagamine Y. Transcriptional regulation of the plasminogen activator inhibitor type 1—With an emphasis on negative regulation. Thrombosis and Haemostasis. 2008;**100**(12):1007-1014. DOI: 10.1160/th08-05-0294

[11] Narayan E, Sawyer G, Parisella S. Faecal glucocorticoid metabolites and body temperature in Australian merino ewes (*Ovis aries*) during summer artificial insemination (AI) program. PLoS One. 2018;**13**(1). DOI: 10.1371/journal.pone.0191961

[12] Bloemhof S, van der Waaij E, Merks J, Knol E. Sow line differences in heat stress tolerance expressed in reproductive performance traits. Journal of Animal Science. 2008;**86**(12):3330-3337. DOI: 10.2527/jas.2008-0862

[13] Australian Wool Innovation. AWI Strategic Plan 2016-2019. 2015. Retrieved from: https://www.wool.com/globalassets/start/about-awi/publications/awi-strategic-plan-2016-19.pdf

[14] Australian Bureau of Statistics. 7121.0-Agricultural Commodities, Australia, 2014-15. 2016. Retrieved from: http://www.abs.gov.au/AUSSTATS/abs@.nsf/Lookup/7121.0Main+Features102014-15?OpenDocument

[15] Australian Wool Innovation. Australian Wool Production Forecast Report December 2017-Wool.com. Australian Wool Innovation. 2017.

Retrieved from: https://www.wool.com/market-intelligence/wool-production-forecasts/australian-wool-production-forecast-report-december-2017/?year=0&month=0&page=1

[16] Australian Bureau of Statistics. 7121.0-Agricultural Commodities, Australia, 2016-17. 2018. Retrieved from: http://www.abs.gov.au/ausstats/abs@.nsf/Latestproducts/7121.0Main%20Features612016-17?opendocument&tabname=Summary&prodno=7121.0&issue=2016-17&num=&view=

[17] Meat and Livestock Australia. Fast Facts - Sheep Industry 2017. 2017. Retrieved from: https://www.mla.com.au/globalassets/mla-corporate/prices--markets/documents/trends--analysis/fast-facts--maps/mla_sheep-fast-facts-2017_final.pdf

[18] Australian Climate Change Science Programme (ACCSP). Australian Climate Change Science Programme. 2016. Retrieved from: http://www.cawcr.gov.au/projects/Climatechange

[19] Meat and Livestock Australia. MLA sheep flock and cattle herd population changes. 2019. Retrieved from: https://www.mla.com.au/globalassets/mla-corporate/prices--markets/documents/trends--analysis/fast-facts--maps/cattle-herd--sheep-flock---population-changes.pdf

[20] Bernabucci U, Lacetera N, Baumgard L, Rhoads R, Ronchi B, Nardone A. Metabolic and hormonal acclimation to heat stress in domesticated ruminants. Animal. 2010;**4**(07):1167-1183. DOI: 10.1017/s175173111000090x

[21] Sejian V. Climate change: Impact on production and reproduction, adaptation mechanisms and mitigation strategies in small ruminants: A review. The Indian Journal of Small Ruminants. 2013;**19**(1):1-21

[22] Intergovernmental Panel on Climate Change (IPCC: AR4). The Intergovernmental Panel on Climate Change 4th Assessment Report. 2007. Available from: http://www.ipcc.ch/publications_and_data/publications_and_data_reports.htm2Google Scholar

[23] NASA Earth Observatory. Global Warming. 2010. Retrieved from: https://earthobservatory.nasa.gov/Features/GlobalWarming/page2.php

[24] CSIRO and the Bureau of Meteorology. Australian Climate Change Science Program; Australia's Changing Climate. 2016. Retrieved from: https://www.climatechangeinaustralia.gov.au/media/ccia/2.1.6/cms_page_media/176/AUSTRALIAS_CHANGING_CLIMATE_1.pdf

[25] Bureau of Meteorology (Australia). State of the Climate 2016: Bureau of Meteorology. 2016. Retrieved from: http://www.bom.gov.au/state-of-the-climate/

[26] Howden S, Crimp S, Stokes C. Climate change and Australian livestock systems: Impacts, research and policy issues. Australian Journal of Experimental Agriculture. 2008;**48**(7):780-788. DOI: 10.1071/ea08033

[27] Sejian V, Lal R, Lakritz J, Ezeji T. Measurement and prediction of enteric methane emission. International Journal of Biometeorology. 2010;**55**(1):1-16. DOI: 10.1007/s00484-010-0356-7

[28] Howden S, Hall W, Bruget D. Heat stress and beef cattle in Australian rangelands: Recent trends and climate change. In: Eldridge D, Freudenberger D, editors. People and Rangelands:

Building the Future. Proceedings of the VI International Rangeland Congress, vol. 6(1). Aitkenvale: International Rangelands Congress Inc.; 1999. pp. 43-45

[29] Sawyer G, Webster D, Narayan E. Measuring wool cortisol and progesterone levels in breeding maiden Australian merino sheep (Ovis aries). PLoS One. 2019;**14**(4). DOI: 10.1371/journal.pone.0214734

[30] Buffington DE, Collazo-Arochu A, Canton HH, Pritt D, Thatcher WW, Collier RJ. Black globe-humidity index (BGHI) as comfort equation for cows. Transactions of the ASAE. 1981;**24**(3):0711-0714. DOI: 10.13031/2013.34325

[31] Campbell P, Pottinger T, Sumpter J. Stress reduces the quality of gametes produced by Rainbow Trout1. Biology of Reproduction. 1992;**47**(6):1140-1150. DOI: 10.1095/biolreprod47.6.1140

[32] Silanikove N. Effects of water scarcity and hot environment on appetite and digestion in ruminants: A review. Livestock Production Science. 1992;**30**:175-194. DOI: 10.1016/S0301-6226(06)80009-6

[33] Belhadj Slimen I, Najar T, Ghram A, Abdrrabba M. Heat stress effects on livestock: Molecular, cellular and metabolic aspects, a review. Journal of Animal Physiology and Animal Nutrition. 2015;**100**(3):401-412. DOI: 10.1111/jpn.12379

[34] Dash S, Chakravarty AK, Singh A, Upadhyay A, Singh M, Yousuf S. Effect of heat stress on reproductive performances of dairy cattle and buffaloes: A review. Veterinary World. 2016;**9**(3):235-244. DOI: 10.14202/vetworld.2016.235-244

[35] Hansen PJ. Exploitation of genetic and physiological determinants of embryonic resistance to elevated temperature to improve embryonic survival in dairy cattle during heat stress. Theriogenology. 2007, 2007;**68**(1):S242-S249. DOI: 10.1016/j.theriogenology.2007.04.008

[36] Hansen P. To be or not to be—Determinants of embryonic survival following heat shock. Theriogenology. 2007;**68**:S40-S48. DOI: 10.1016/j.theriogenology.2007.03.013

[37] Kapoor A, Leen J, Matthews S. Molecular regulation of the hypothalamic-pituitary-adrenal axis in adult male Guinea pigs after prenatal stress at different stages of gestation. The Journal of Physiology. 2008;**586**(17):4317-4326. DOI: 10.1113/jphysiol.2008.153684

[38] Seckl J, Holmes M. Mechanisms of disease: Glucocorticoids, their placental metabolism and fetal 'programming' of adult pathophysiology. Nature Clinical Practice Endocrinology & Metabolism. 2007;**3**(6):479-488. DOI: 10.1038/ncpendmet0515

[39] Glover V. Prenatal stress and its effects on the fetus and the child: Possible underlying biological mechanisms. In: Perinatal Programming of Neurodevelopment. New York, NY: Springer; 2015. pp. 269-283. DOI: 10.1007/978-1-4939-1372-5_13

[40] Du J, Di HS, Guo L, Li ZH, Wang GL. Hyperthermia causes bovine mammary epithelial cell death by a mitochondrial-induced pathway. Journal of Thermal Biology. 2008;**33**:37-47. DOI: 10.1016/j.jtherbio.2007.06.002

[41] Kijas J, Townley D, Dalrymple B, Heaton M, Maddox J, McGrath A, et al. A genome wide survey of SNP variation reveals the genetic structure of sheep breeds. PLoS One. 2009;**4**(3):e4668. DOI: 10.1371/journal.pone.0004668

[42] Koubkova M, Haertlova H, Knizkova I, Kunc P, Flusser J, Dolezal O. Influence of high environmental temperatures and evaporative cooling on some physiological, hematological and biochemical parameters in high-yielding dairy cows. Czech Journal of Animal Science-UZPI (Czech Republic). 2002:309-318

[43] McDowell RE. Improvement of livestock production in warm climates: Freeman, San Francisco, California, 1972, 711 pp. Livestock Production Science. 1972;**1**(2):225-226

[44] Bianca W. Relative importance of dry- and wet-bulb temperatures in causing heat stress in cattle. Nature. 1962;**195**(4838):251-252. DOI: 10.1038/195251a0

[45] Hayes B, Carrick M, Bowman P, Goddard M. Genotype×environment interaction for milk production of daughters of Australian dairy sires from test-day records. Journal of Dairy Science. 2003;**86**(11):3736-3744. DOI: 10.3168/jds.s0022-0302(03)73980-0

[46] Finocchiaro R, van Kaam J, Portolano B, Misztal I. Effect of heat stress on production of Mediterranean dairy sheep. Journal of Dairy Science. 2005;**88**(5):1855-1864. DOI: 10.3168/jds.s0022-0302(05)72860-5

[47] Horowitz M. From molecular and cellular to integrative heat defence during exposure to chronic heat. Comparative Biochemistry and Physiology Part A. 2002;**131**:475-483. DOI: 10.1016/S1095-6433(01)00500-1

[48] Fuller A, Mitchell D, Maloney S, Hetem R. Towards a mechanistic understanding of the responses of large terrestrial mammals to heat and aridity associated with climate change. Climate Change Responses. 2016;**3-10**(1). DOI: 10.1186/s40665-016-0024-1

[49] Tattersall GJ, Sinclair BJ, Withers PC, Fields PA, Seebacher F, Cooper CE. Coping with thermal challenges: Physiological adaptations to environmental temperatures. Comparative Physiology. 2012;**2**: 2151-2202. DOI: 10.1002/cphy.c110055

[50] Smith S, Edmonds J, Hartin C, Mundra A, Calvin K. Near-term acceleration in the rate of tesmperature change. Nature Climate Change. 2015;**5**(4):333-336. DOI: 10.1038/nclimate2552

[51] West JW. Effects of heat stress on production in dairy cattle. Climate change: Impact on production and reproduction, adaptation mechanisms and mitigation strategies in small ruminants: A review. Journal of Dairy Science. 2003;**86**:2131-2144. Available from: https://www.researchgate.net/publication/259865707/download

[52] Wall E, Wreford A, Topp K, Moran D. Biological and economic consequences heat stress due to a changing climate on UK livestock. Advances in Animal Biosciences. 2010;**1**:53-53. DOI: 10.1017/S2040470010001962

[53] Rooke J, Arnott G, Dwyer C, Rutherford K. The importance of the gestation period for welfare of lambs: Maternal stressors and lamb vigour and wellbeing. The Journal of Agricultural Science. 2014;**153**(03):497-519. DOI: 10.1017/s002185961400077x

[54] Alliston CW, Ulberg LC. Early pregnancy loss in sheep at ambient temperatures of 70° and 90°F as determined by embryo transfer. Journal of Animal Science. 1961;**20**(3):608-613. DOI: 10.2527/jas1961.203608x

[55] Gordon I. Embryo transfer and associated techniques in sheep. In: Controlled Reproduction in Farm Animals Series, Volume 2: Controlled

Reproduction in Sheep and Goats. Oxon, UK: CAB International; 1997

[56] Hansen PJ, Drost M, Rivera RM, Paula-Lopes FF, Al-Katanani YM, Kriniger CE, et al. Adverse impact of heat stress on embryo production: Causes and strategies for mitigation. Theriogenology. 2001;**55**:91-103

[57] Gordon I, Boland MP, McGovern H, Lynn G. Effect of season on superovulatory responses and embryo quality in Holstein cattle in Saudi Arabia. Theriogenology. 1987;**27**(1):231

[58] Naqvi S, Maurya V, Gulyani R, Joshi A, Mittal J. The effect of thermal stress on superovulatory response and embryo production in Bharat merino ewes. Small Ruminant Research. 2004;**55**(1-3):57-63. DOI: 10.1016/j.smallrumres.2004.02.009

[59] United Nations Food Agriculture Organization. Climate Change and Food Security: A Framework Document. 1st ed. Rome, Italy: United Nations Food and Agriculture; 2008. Available from: http://www.fao.org/3/k2595e/k2595e00.pdf

[60] Silanikove N. The physiological basis of adaptation of goats to scarcity of food and water in harsh environments. Small Ruminant Research. 2000;**35**:181-193. DOI: 10.1016/S0921-4488(99)00096-6

[61] Collier RJ, Baumgard LH, Lock AL, Bauman DE. Physiological limitations, nutrient partitioning. In: Sylvester-Bradley R, Wiseman J, editors. Yield of Farmed Species. Constraints and Opportunities in the 21st Century. Nottingham, UK: Nottingham University Press; 2005. pp. 351-377

[62] Gaughan JB, Lacetera N, Valtorta SE, Khalifa HH, Hahn L, Mader T. Response of domestic animals to climate challenges. In: Ebi KL, Burton I, McGregor GR, editors. Biometeorology of Adaptation to Climate Variability and Change. Heidelberg, Germany: Springer Science; 2009. pp. 131-170

[63] Khalifa HH, Shalaby T, Abdel-Khalek TMM. An approach to develop a biometeorological thermal discomfort index for sheep and goats under Egyptian conditions. In: Proceeding of the 17th International Congress of Biometeorology (International Society of Biometeorology). Garmisch-Partenkirchen, Germany: Offenbach am Main; 2005. pp. 118-122

[64] Horowitz M, Kaspler P, Marmary Y, Oron Y. Evidence for contribution of effector organ cellular responses to biphasic dynamics of heat acclimation. Journal of Applied Physiology. 1996;**80**:77-85. DOI: 10.1152/jappl.1996.80.1.77

[65] Hahn GL. Dynamic responses of cattle to thermal heat load. Journal of Animal Science. 1999;**77**(suppl. 2):10-20

[66] Horowitz M. Heat acclimation: Phenotypic plasticity and cues to the underlying molecular mechanisms. Journal of Thermal Biology. 2001;**26**:357-363. DOI: 10.1016/S0306-4565(01)00044-4

[67] Maloyan A, Palmon A, Horowitz M. Heat acclimation increases the basal Hsp72 level and alters its production dynamics during heat stress. American Journal of Physiology–Regulatory, Integrative and Comparative Physiology. 1999;**276**:R1506-R1515. DOI: 10.1152/ajpregu.1999.276.5.R1506

[68] Bernabucci U, Bani P, Ronchi B, Lacetera N, Nardone A. Influence of short and long-term exposure to a hot environment on rumen passage rate and diet digestibility in Friesian heifers. Journal of Dairy Science. 1999;**82**:967-973. DOI: 10.3168/jds.S0022-0302(99)75316-6

[69] Mittal JP, Ghosh PK. Body temperature, respiration rate ad

pulse rate in Corriedale, Marwari and Magra sheep in the Rajasthan desert. The Journal of Agricultural Science. 1979;**39**:587-591. DOI: 10.1017/S0021859600038995

[70] Ferguson MB, Thompson AN, Gordon DJ, Hyder MW, Kearney GA, Oldham CM, et al. The wool production and reproduction of merino ewes can be predicted from changes in liveweight during pregnancy and lactation. Animal Production Science. 2011;**51**:763-775. DOI: 10.1071/AN10158

[71] Wu G, Bazer F, Wallace J, Spencer T. Board-invited review: Intrauterine growth retardation: Implications for the animal sciences. Journal of Animal Science. 2006;**84**(9):2316-2337. DOI: 10.2527/jas.2006-156

[72] Rhoads ML, Rhoads RP, Van Baale MJ, Collier RJ, Sanders SR, Weber WJ, et al. Effects of heat stress and plane of nutrition on lactating Holstein cows: I. Production, metabolism and aspects of circulating somatotropin. Journal of Dairy Science. 2009;**92**:1986-1997. DOI: 10.3168/jds.2008-1641

[73] Schwartz G, Rhoads ML, Van Baale MJ, Rhoads RP, Baumgard LH. Effects of a supplemental yeast culture on heat-stressed lactating Holstein cows. Journal of Dairy Science. 2009;**92**:935-942. DOI: 10.3168/jds.2008-1496

[74] Drackley JK. Biology of dairy cows during the transition period: The final frontier. Journal of Dairy Science. 1999;**82**:2259-2273. DOI: 10.3168/jds.S0022-0302(99)75474-3

[75] Yousef MK. Measurements of heat production and heat loss. In: Yousef MK, editor. Stress Physiology in Livestock, Vol. 1. Basic Principles. Boca Raton, FL, USA: CRC Press; 1985. pp. 35-46

[76] Hahn GM. Hyperthermia and Cancer. New York: Plenium Press; 1982. pp. 74-85

[77] Streffer C. Aspect of metabolic change in hyperthermia. Recent Results in Cancer Research. 1988;**197**:7-43

[78] Higashikubo R, White RA, Roti Roti JL. Flow cytometric Brd Urdpulse-chase study of heat induced cellcycle progression delays. Cell Proliferation. 1993;**26**:337-348

[79] Plant JW. Field investigations into reproductive wastage in sheep. Refresher Course for Veterinarians Proceedings. 1981;**58**:411-440

[80] Refshauge G, Brien F, Hinch G, van de Ven R. Neonatal lamb mortality: Factors associated with the death of Australian lambs. Animal Production Science. 2016;**56**(4):726-735. DOI: 10.1071/an15121

[81] Behrendt R, van Burgel AJ, Bailey A, Barber P, Curnow M, Gordon DJ, et al. On-farm paddock scale comparisons across southern Australia confirm that increasing the nutrition of Merino ewes improves their production and the lifetime performance of their progeny. Animal Production Science. 2011;**51**:805-812. DOI: 10.1071/AN10183

[82] Allworth MB, Wrigley HA, Cowling A. Fetal and lamb losses from pregnancy scanning to lamb marking in commercial sheep flocks in southern New South Wales. Animal Production Science. 2016;**57**:2060-2065. DOI: 10.1071/AN16166

[83] Wolfenson D, Roth Z, Meidan R. Impaired reproduction in heat-stressed cattle: Basic and applied aspects. Animal Reproduction Science. 2000;**60-61**:535-547. DOI: 10.1016/S0378-4320(00)00102-0

[84] Ulberg LC, Burfening PJ. Embryo death resulting from adverse environment on spermatozoa or ova. Journal of Animal Science. 1967;**26**(3):571-577. DOI: 10.2527/jas1967.263571x

[85] Lindsay DR, Knight TW, Smith JF, Oldham CM. Studies in ovine fertility inagricultural regions of Western Australia: Ovulation rate, fertility and lambing performance. Australian Journal Agricultural Research. 1975;**26**:189-198. DOI: 10.1071/AR9750189

[86] Kleemann DO, Walker SK. Fertility in South Australian commercial Merino flocks: Relationships between reproductive traits and environmental cues. Theriogenology. 2005;**63**:2416-2433. DOI: 10.1016/j.theriogenology.2004.09.052

[87] Yates D. Measurement of physiological stress response, effects of stress on reproduction, and management practices for avoiding embryonic wastage [PhD thesis]. New Mexico State University; 2009

[88] Roberts RM, Bazer FW, Thatcher WW. Biochemical interactions between blastocysts and endometrium in the large domestic animals. Journal of Biosciences. 1984;**2**:63-74. DOI: 10.1007/BF02716717

[89] Piper LR, Bindon BM, Atkins KD, Mcguirk BJ. Genetic variation in ovulation rate in merino ewes aged 18 months. Proceedings of the Australian Society of Animal Production. 1980;**13**:409-412

[90] Owen J, Crees S, Williams J, Davies D. Prolificacy and 50-day lamb weight of ewes in the Cambridge sheep breed. Animal Science. 1986;**42**(3):355-363. DOI: 10.1017/S0003356100018134

[91] Morley FHW, White DH, Kenney PA, Davis IF. Predicting ovulation rate from the live weight in ewes. Agricultural Systems. 1978;**3**:27-45. DOI: 10.1016/0308-521X(78)90004-5

[92] Kelly RW, Thompson KF, Hawker H, Crosbie SF, McEwan JC. Liveweight, ovulation rate and wool growth responses of light and heavy ewes to differential feeding. New Zealand Journal of Experimental Agriculture. 1983;**11**:219-224. DOI: 10.1071/AN10158

[93] Thompson KF, Crosbie SF, Kelly RW, McEwan JC. The effect of liveweight and liveweight change on ewe ovulation rate at 3 oestrus cycles. New Zealand Journal of Agricultural Research. 1985;**28**:457-462. DOI: 10.1080/00288233.1985.10417990

[94] Borg R, Notter D, Kott R. Genetic analysis of ewe stayability and its association with lamb growth and adult production. Journal of Animal Science. 2009;**87**(11):3515-3524. DOI: 10.2527/jas.2008-1623

[95] McCrabb GJ, McDonald BJ, Hennoste LM. Lamb birthweight in sheep differently acclimatized to a hot environment. Australian Journal of Agricultural Research. 1993;**44**(5):933-943. DOI: 10.1017/S0021859600074311

[96] Khodaei-Motlagh M, Shahneh AZ, Masoumi R, Derensis F. Alterations in reproductive hormones during heat stress in dairy cattle. African Journal of Biotechnology. 2011;**10**(29):5552-5558

[97] Brien F, Cloete S, Fogarty N, Greeff J, Hebart M, Hiendleder S, et al. A review of the genetic and epigenetic factors affecting lamb survival. Animal Production Science. 2014;**54**(6):667-693. DOI: 10.1071/an13140

[98] Marai IFM, El-Darawany AA, Fadiel A, Abdel-Hafez MAM. Physiological traits as affected by heat stress in sheep—A review. Small Ruminant Research. 2007;**71**(1-3):1-12. DOI: 10.1016/j.smallrumres.2006.10.003

[99] Dobson H, Smith R. What is stress, and how does it affect reproduction? Animal Reproduction Science. 2000;**60-61**:743-752. DOI: 10.1016/s0378-4320(00)00080-4

[100] Wolfenson D, Lew BJ, Thatcher WW, Graber Y, Meidan R. Seasonal and acute heat stress effects on steroid production by dominant follicles in cows. Animal Reproduction Science. 1997;**47**(1-2):9-19. DOI: 10.1016/S0378-4320(96)01638-7

[101] De Rensis F, Scaramuzzi RJ. Heat stress and seasonal effects on reproduction in the dairy cow—A review. Theriogenology. 2003;**60**(6):1139-1151. DOI: 10.1016/S0093-691X(03)00126-2

[102] Crimp SJ, Stokes CJ, Howden SM, Moore AD, Jacobs B, Brown PR, et al. Managing Murray–Darling basin livestock systems in a variable and changing climate: Challenges and opportunities. The Rangeland Journal. 2010;**32**:293-304. DOI: 10.1071/RJ10039

Chapter 5

Endocrinology of Reproduction in Crustaceans

Ramachandra Reddy Pamuru

Abstract

Crustaceans have become the most popular proteinacious foods to meet the food demand of ever growing human population in the World. But, the culturing of crustacean species has many problems, including limited availability of quality seed. Out of all conventional methods practiced to increase seed of good quality and quantity, manipulation of the endocrine system of brood stock is found to be one of the best methods. Regulation of crustacean reproduction is under the control of many hormones and factors. The eyestalk hormones, namely gonad/vitellogenin-inhibiting hormone (VIH) and mandibular organ inhibiting hormone (MOIH) show negative effects on maturation, whereas the other eyestalk hormones show mixed effects on maturation. The non-eyestalk hormones namely gonad stimulating hormone (GSH), methyl farnesoate (MF) and ecdysteroids are ovarian maturation inducers in crustaceans. The pros and cons of endocrine manipulation in crustaceans are discussed in this chapter.

Keywords: crustaceans, endocrine hormones, regulation of reproduction

1. Introduction

Crustaceans, a major group of animals which serve as food for humans and animals come under phylum Arthropoda. There are about 45,000 crustacean species distributed throughout the World. The crab, marine shrimps, crayfishes, lobsters and freshwater prawns are edible and they belong to crustacea. This group of animals is free-living and the habitat of most of them is freshwater or marine, where few of them are semi terrestrial. Edible crustaceans have lots of importance because of its role in acting as rich protein food, sustainability in culturing and trading. They possess significant economic value in Nations of developing which undoubtedly provide food security in both the production and transportation to within and to other Nations. The acceptance of crustacean food in World has also increased due to its softness, flavor, easy digestion and numerous health benefits due to the presence of protein, minerals and vitamins which are known to prevent a range of diseases. The seafood, especially crustacean proteinacious food is famous in many countries and has its own demand. Most of crustacean food is produced in China and other Asian countries. The fresh, the frozen and the snacks are different forms of crustacean food available throughout the World, supplied from the food industry. Besides food industry, other major industries that use crustaceans are pharmaceutical and cosmetic industries. The crustacean pigments and natural compounds of shell are holding high value in the cosmetic industry. Globally, the edible crustacean production is about 10 million tons per year through fisheries and aquaculture farming. Due to its significance, the crustacean World market has reached to US $ 147 in the year 2017 and is anticipated to grow at a reasonable rate in the years to follow. Though the crustacean production is increasing steadily in the global market, it is not at a great rate to meet the demands of the ever growing human population on the globe. Due to several reasons, crustacean aquaculture industry is facing numerous troubles in obtaining expected productivity. One of such reasons is limited availability of good quality seed, a potential startup for high yield of protein.

Crustaceans are mostly unisexual and can be easily distinguished into the male and female by morphology. Male and female reproductive organs are developed to produce and reproduce young ones in the brood sack of the female. The usage of quality seed is a key to get increased productivity of the quality protein in aquaculture. Naturally captured crustacean seed is found the most promising one to get more protein through culture. But, the availability of seed in the nature is limited and tedious to obtain. To overcome this, a classical eyestalk ablation method is introduced to induce spawning in the brood stock [1]. Removal of eyestalk climi nates the synthesis and release of eyestalk gonad inhibitory principle from neurohemal X-organ sinus gland complex, which promotes maturation [2]. Because of cautery of eyestalk, this method causes the highest mortality in the brood stock and loss of hemolymph very often leads to production of inferior quality seed. In search of an alternative, the researchers are working in multiple directions to get quality seed. Among all, the endocrine manipulation of crustacean hormones is one of the best methods for quality seed production.

2. Maturation and hormones

The proper maturation of gonads in crustacea provides the quality seed production. The maturation in crustaceans happens mainly due to activation of biosynthesis of female reproductive egg protein called vitellogenin. Vitellogenin is a lipoprotein used for the nourishment (energy requirement) of developing embryo. The site of vitellogenesis in crustaceans is various tissues, including the ovary. The major sites for vitellogenesis are ovary, hepatopancreas and epidermis. Most of the crabs are holding hepatopancreas as vitellogenin synthesizing site whereas in other crustaceans, it is epidermis or hepatopancreas along with the ovary. In natural maturation vitellogenin is produced as pre-vitellogenin and it undergoes cleavage to produce the mature vitellogenin/vitellin molecules of bearing different molecular sizes. The size and number of vitellins varies from one species to other. These vitellins via hemolymph are transported to ovary and they deposit in the developing oocytes. The accumulation of vitellin in the developing ovary is continued until the ovary reaches to fully matured stage [3]. The female reproductive protein vitellin/vitellogenin is a good indicator of reproductive activity in crustaceans and is frequently used to determine the regulatory functions of endocrine hormones [4].

There are many factors that regulate the maturation of ovary in crustacean brood stock. The eyestalk neural tissue in crustacea secrets a number of neuroendocrine hormones and is analogous to vertebrate pituitary-hypothalamus. The vitellogenesis/gonad-inhibiting hormone (VIH/GIH), mandibular organ-inhibiting hormone (MOIH), crustacean hyperglycemic hormone (CHH), molt-inhibiting hormone (MIH), biogenic amines and opioids are the major secretory products of eyestalk. These eyestalk products play a crucial role in regulating the maturation in crustaceans. The products of Y-organs and mandibular organs called ecdysteroids and methyl farnesoate (MF) respectively and gonad stimulating hormone (GSH) are non-eyestalk hormones involved in the regulation of ovarian maturation [5, 6].

Besides these, the ovarian maturation is also regulated by the external factors such as temperature, salinity, pH, food availability in the pond and heavy metals present in the water through endocrine regulation. However, the regulation of reproduction is a complex process in crustacea and its understanding requires the detailed description of action of internal and external factors.

3. Factors involved in the regulation of reproduction

Endocrine hormones such as eyestalk neuropeptides, GSH, opioids, biogenic amines, ecdysteroids and MF are endogenous factors that regulate reproduction in crustaceans [6]. The internal factors are of two types based on their action in the regulation of reproduction. Hormones which promote reproduction come under "positive regulators", whereas those that suppress the reproduction are called "negative regulators". The positive regulators are MF, ecdysteroids and GSH, and the negative regulators are VIH/GIH and MOIH. Some factors like CHH, MIH, biogenic amines and opioids are found to be having both the actions. The Y-organs, mandibular organs, brain, thoracic ganglia and ovary are responsible for the release of a variety of reproductive regulatory hormones and factors beside the major endocrine centers of the eyestalks. The role of these hormones and factors in the regulation of crustacean maturation, especially in the ovarian growth is discussed here.

3.1 Factors of X-organ sinus gland complex

The eyestalk neural tissue is divided into medulla extern interna and terminalis. Neural clusters located in these three parts of neural tissue are responsible for the secretion of all eyestalk peptide hormones and other factors. These secretions are initially stored in a neurohemal organ sinus gland located in the eyestalk and it finally secretes into the stream of hemolymph to show its action at the target tissue. The eyestalk neural tissue, cluster of neuronal cells and sinus gland are collectively called "neurohemal X-organ sinus gland complex". The hormones of eyestalk such as CHH, VIH, MIH, MOIH and other peptides are collectively called as CHH-family peptides. These peptide hormones are classified as Type I and II based on the presence or absence of Glycine residue at 12th position of their mature peptides [7]. The secretions of eyestalk are as follows and are discussed in Section 3.1.1.

3.1.1 Vitellogenesis/gonad-inhibiting hormone

The prime role of eyestalk GIH/VIH in crustacea is inhibition of ovarian/gonad maturation. Panouse [1] first identified the presence of GIH in *Palaemon* (*Leander*) *serratus* (*P. serratus*). He founded the speedy rise in size of ovary and precocious egg deposition in the ovaries by the removal of eyestalk gonad inhibitory factor (GIH) from immature *P. serratus*. Later the same was reported in other crustacean species (See review [3, 8]). Since the lack of exact bioassay, identification and characterization of VIH neuropeptides the literature available is limited. However, VIH was identified and characterized in a variety of crustaceans. The ovarian fragments of *Procambarus bouvieri* were incubated *in vitro* with isolated VIH from the same species and inhibition of vitellogenin m-RNA levels were found in ovarian fragments [9]. Soyez et al. [10] first reported the complete structure of VIH in American lobster, *Homarus americanus* (*H. americanus*), and later Gréve et al. [11] in the terrestrial isopod *Armadillidium vulgare*.

In the recent past, recombinant proteins were identified as potential molecules for altering the biological functions. The recombinant GIH/VIH protein was synthesized for a variety of crustaceans. The r-GIH was synthesized for lobster *Nephrops norvegicus* and using this identified the GIH synthesizing cells in eyestalk neural tissue [12]. The VIH activity of secondary structure of *H. americanus* recombinant VIH (rHoa-VIH) which was assured by bacterial expression system was incubated with *Marsupenaeus japonicus* (*M. japonicus*) ovarian fragments *in vitro* [13]. Ohira et al. [13] was tested the reduced vitellogenin m-RNA levels in the ovary of *M. japonicus* incubated with c-terminus amidated rHoa-VIH. Advancement of technology reveals the gene function and is not restricted to characterize the crustacean genes. The gene –silencing using RNAi methodology is in use to silence the inhibitory CHH-family peptides, to activate reproduction and growth in crustaceans. VIH gene silencing was demonstrated in *Penaeus monodon* (*P. monodon*). The *in vivo* functional gene silencing of *P. monodon* VIH (Pem-VIH) with increased vitellogenin m-RNA levels was reported by administration of Pem-VIH ds m-RNA [14].

Though the mechanism of VIH/GIH induced inhibition of reproduction is not clear, from the available literature, it is identified that VIH shows its action in two intracellular signaling pathways in the ovary such as a) cyclic nucleotide signaling and b) calcium ion and protein kinase C signaling [15]. In one way, VIH induces its inhibitory action by activating the cyclic nucleotides adenylyl cyclase or guanylyl cyclase or both (**Figure 1**). Binding of VIH to G protein receptor activates the G protein which activates adenylyl cyclase that produce cAMP from ATP. On the other hand VIH may also stimulate the guanylyl cyclase through its receptors (GCR)

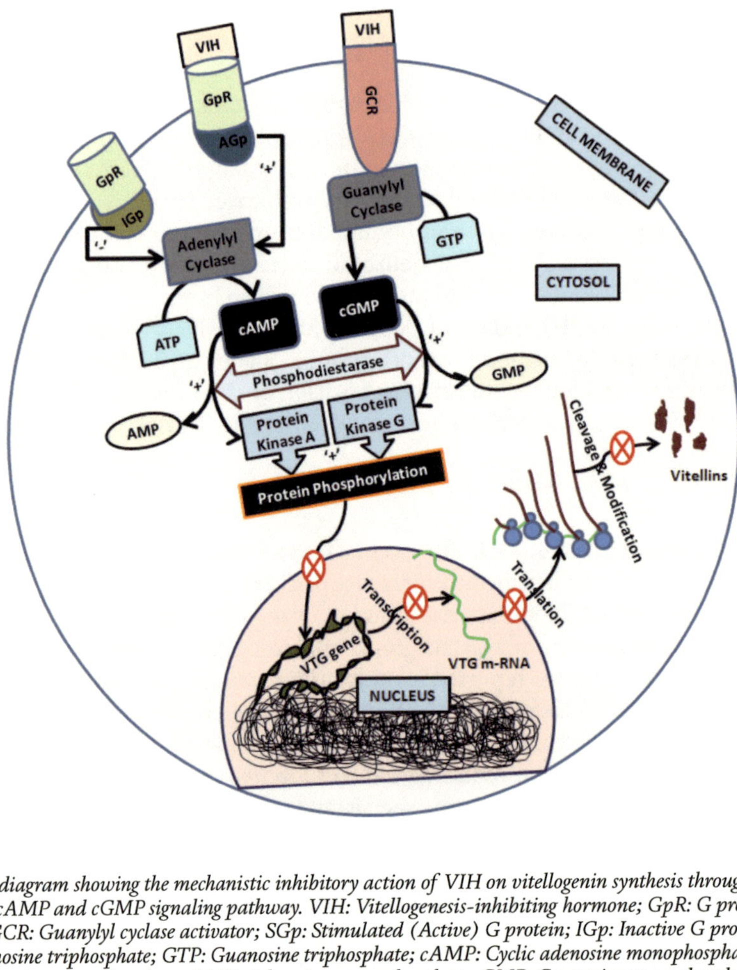

Figure 1.
Schematic diagram showing the mechanistic inhibitory action of VIH on vitellogenin synthesis through secondary messenger cAMP and cGMP signaling pathway. VIH: Vitellogenesis-inhibiting hormone; GpR: G protein receptor; GCR: Guanylyl cyclase activator; SGp: Stimulated (Active) G protein; IGp: Inactive G protein; ATP: Adenosine triphosphate; GTP: Guanosine triphosphate; cAMP: Cyclic adenosine monophosphate; cGMP: Cyclic guanosine monophosphate; AMP: Adenosine monophosphate; GMP: Guanosine monophosphate; VTG: Vitellogenin; '+' and '-' denotes activation and inhibition respectively; ⊗: supression of the reaction.

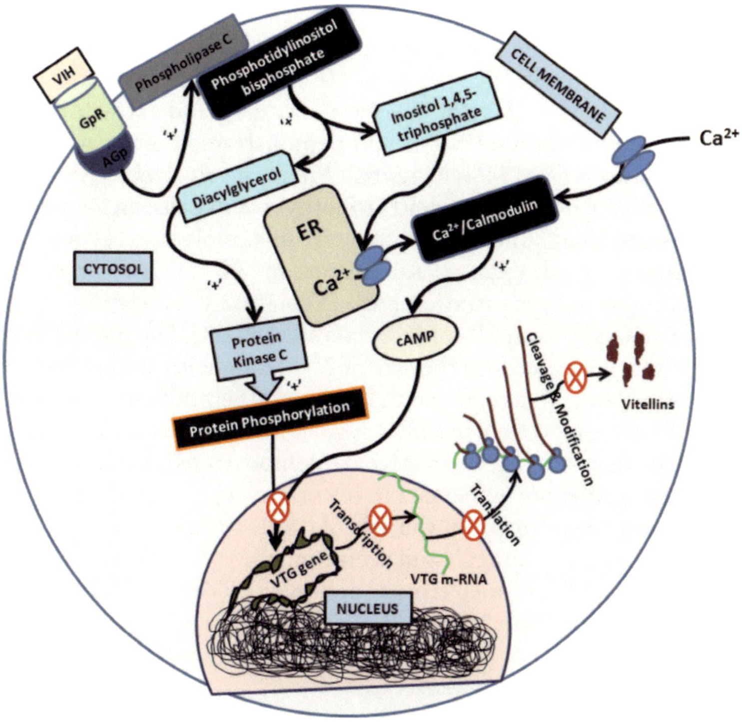

Figure 2.
Schematic diagram showing the mechanistic inhibitory action of VIH on vitellogenin synthesis through Ca^{2+} and protein kinase C signaling pathway. VIH: Vitellogenesis-inhibiting hormone; GpR: G protein receptor; AGp: Active G protein; cAMP: Cyclic adenosine monophosphate; ER: Endoplasmic reticulum; Ca^{2+}: Calcium ion; VTG: Vitellogenin; '+' and '-' denotes activation and inhibition respectively; ⊗: the negetive regulation.

which leads to conversion of GTP into cGMP. Both the cyclic nucleotides by the action of phosphodiesterase activate protein kinase A and G respectively for cAMP and cGMP. Increased protein phosphorylation induced by protein kinase A or G or both suppresses the gene expression of vitellogenin in the nucleus, thereby reduces the vitellogenin protein levels in the ovarian follicles [16].

Figure 2 explains the second mechanistic action of VIH inhibitory pathway through activation of protein kinase C by diacylglycerol, inosital and calcium ions (calmodulin). The high titer of circulatory VIH, binds to G protein receptors (GpR) in the developing ovarian follicles. Upon binding of GpR with VIH, activates the G protein, which initiates the conversion of phosphotidyl bisphosphate into diacylglycerol and inositol 1, 4, 5 – triphosphate upon activation of phoshpolipase C. The diacylglycerol activates the protein phosphorylation through protein kinase C. On the other hand inositol 1, 4, 5 – triphosphate induces the increase of intracellular free calcium (Ca^{2+}) from the endoplasmic reticulum in addition to the calcium available through calcium transported from the extracellular space to cytosol. Calmodulin bound or free Ca^{2+} activates the synthesis of cAMP, which directly inhibits the gene expression of vitellogenin gene in the nucleus along with high levels of protein phosphorylation [16].

3.1.2 Mandibular organ-inhibiting hormone

The MOIH, an eyestalk neuropeptide known negative regulator of reproduction is identified in many crustaceans [17]. More specifically, mandibular organs (MOs) involved in maturation of crustaceans through its secretory product methyl farnesoate are under negative control of MOIH. The elevated MF levels of 54.1 and 106.9 ng/gland in MO are reported respectively, after unilateral and bilateral eyestalk ablation respectively in *H. americanus* [18]. In the same study the suppressed MF levels are recorded in MOs after injection of sinus gland extracts to bilateral eyestalk ablated *H. americanus*. Chaves [19] demonstrated the negative effect of MOIH on MF synthesis from MO in crayfish *Procambarus clarkii (P. clarkii)* by measuring the activity of farnesoic acid O-methyl transferase an enzyme involved in MF synthesis and also found 20–100 fold rise in hemolymph MF levels during 8th–12th day after eyestalk ablation. An increase in MO size is also recorded in *H. americanus* during ovarian maturation [20]. Premature vitellogenesis is observed in juvenile *Libinia emarginata* after MO implantation [21]. During the ovarian maturation process an increase in the size of MO along with an increase in ovarian index and oocyte diameter is reported in the natural reproductive cycle of crab *Oziothelphusa senex senex* (*O. senex senex*) [22]. Direct studies showing the MOIH action against the release of MF from MO are demonstrated in many studies. The above mentioned studies are evidenced in the stimulatory role of MO and MF in crustacean reproduction. However, the role of MOIH in the regulation of reproduction by inhibiting the synthesis and secretion of MF from MO is clear from the limited literature, but the mechanistic action of MOIH is not clear and further studies are needed to establish it.

3.1.3 Crustacean hyperglycemic hormone

The major CHH-family peptide synthesized and released from the eyestalk neural tissue is a crustacean hyperglycemic hormone (CHH). The onset of vitellogenesis is regulated by CHH besides its principal activity in carbohydrate metabolism [23]. Studies on CHH regulated reproduction are limited. At first, the role of CHH-A and CHH-B on reproduction is demonstrated in *H. americanus* [9, 23]. De Kleijn et al. [24] has found that the onset of vitellogenin synthesis is triggered by Hoa-CHH-A and oocyte development in late stages of maturation is by Hoa-CHH-B. Similarly, in *Metapenaeus ensis* (*M. ensis*) isolated two CHH-family peptides involved in ovarian development, especially in early stage (CHH-A) and, middle and later stage (CHH-B) [25]. In contrast, *in vitro* inhibition of vitellogenin and its expression in *Penaeus semisulcatus* ovarian fragments by *Penaeus japonicus* CHH are reported [26].

The isoforms of CHH may be received by different types of receptors responsible for a variety of physiological functions including reproduction. It is evidenced through occurrence of CHH receptors on the membrane of Y-organs the principle glands synthesize ecdysteroids in *Carcinus maenas* (*C. maenas*) and *Gecarcinus lateralis* [27, 28]. The recombinant CHH reduced 51% of ecdysteroid levels from Y-organs of crab *C. maenas* [27]. Since CHH isoforms are showing similarity with other CHH-family peptides and its pleiotropic nature, they might display functions of important depends on the tissue they reach. Due to the CHH importance in crustacean reproduction and endocrine manipulation, further mechanistic actions are necessary to elucidate.

3.1.4 Molt-inhibiting hormone

Molt inhibition is the fundamental role of eyestalk MIH. Through inhibiting the synthesis and secretion of molting hormone (ecdysteroids) from Y-organs (molting glands) MIH regulates molting. Due to its pleiotropic nature, MIH is reported for its involvement in the onset of vitellogenesis in crustaceans. The MIH mediated reproduction is not very clear and reports are showing both positive and negative effects on maturation. The concealed onset of vitellogenesis by MIH is identified in shrimp

M. ensis [29]. In the same species also reported recombinant Me-MIH-B induced vitellogenin expression in ovary and hepatopancreas in a dose dependent manner *in vitro*. Recent studies identified and characterized the hepatopancreatic MIH binding proteins in maturing female crab *Callinectes sapidus* (*C. sapidus*) [30]. Zmora et al. [30] Identified high cAMP (a secondary messenger) levels in hepatopancreatic tissue incubated with *C. sapidus* MIH and predicted the mechanistic action of MIH in the onset of reproduction. Zmora et al. [30] reported the dynamics of MIH during different stages of ovarian maturation in *C. sapidus*. They reported the antagonistic action of MIH on growth (inhibition) and reproduction (induction) by comparing the MIH titers at premature (low) and mature stages (four fold higher) of ovary. Moreover, the gonad stimulatory effect of MIH-B isolated from *M. ensis* is tested and its pattern of expression in eyestalk neural tissue is correlated with ovarian maturation cycle [31]. Tiu and Chan [29] found elevated hemolymph and ovarian vitellogenin protein levels along with hepatopancreatic and ovarian vitellogenin m-RNA levels upon administration with Me-MIH-B *in vivo*. The ds-RNA of Me-MIH-B injection concealed the vitellogenin m-RNA levels in hepatopancreas and ovary along with lowered vitellogenin protein levels in hemolymph and ovary in *M. ensis* [29]. However, the growth and reproduction are antagonistic in crabs and sequential in prawns and shrimps. Furthermore, studies are immensely needed on MIH for manipulation of crustacean reproduction in order to uphold sustainable aquaculture.

3.1.5 Opioid peptides

Small peptides containing five amino acid residues released from eyestalks are called opioids. Their presence is well defined in vertebrates [32] and is also reported in a few invertebrates including crustaceans using modern techniques like radioimmunoassay (RIA), high performance liquid chromatography (HPLC) and immunohistochemistry (IHC). In crustaceans, opioids are identified in the eyestalk neural tissue and are released from sinus glands into the hemolymph. The endogenous opioids found in crustaceans are named as leucine-enkephalin and methionine-enkephalin. Limited reports are available for opioids induced reproduction in crustaceans [33]. The *in vivo* experiment was conducted to investigate the role of endogenous opioids on reproduction in crab *Uca pugilator*. Whereas, observed dose dependent inhibition of ovarian development by injecting methionine-enkephalin. In *P. clarkii*, it is proved that incubation of thoracic ganglion alone with ovarian fragments *in vitro* does not cause any change in the ovary, whereas incubation along with methionine-enkephalin reduced the ovarian maturation in a dose dependent manner [34]. Out of two enkephalins identified, only leucin-enkehpalin is found to be involved in the regulation of maturation in prawn *Penaeus indicus* (*P. indicus*) [35]. The induction of maturation by leucine-enkephalin is tested in *P. indicus* and *O. senex senex* [34, 35]. However, the role of opioids in crustaceans is controversial and is required to conduct more studies to determine its specific mechanistic action and use in endocrine manipulation of reproduction.

3.1.6 Biogenic amines

In decapods, biogenic amines are well reported as regulators of reproduction. Initially these amines act as neuroregulators and later as neurohormones. They play an important role in synthesis and releasing of endocrine hormones involved in the regulation of reproduction [36]. The hormones like CHH-family peptides (GIH, CHH, MIH, RPDH and BPDH) and GSH are influenced by biogenic amines [37]. The identified biogenic amines in crustaceans are serotonin (5-hydroxy tryptamine; 5-HT) and dopamine, and they influence the ovarian maturation (**Table 1**).

S.no.	Crustacean species	Biogenic amine and its function	References
1	*Oziothelphusa senex senex*	Serotonin—stimulates ovarian index and oocyte size	Sainath et al. [38]
2	*Ucca pugilator*	5-HT—gonadal development and maturation; stimulates release of GSH Dopamine—stimulates the testicular maturation	Sarojini et al. [39]; Richardson et al. [37]
3	*Fenneropenaeus merguiensis*	5-HT—female gonadal maturation	Makkapan et al. [40]
4	*Litopenaeus vannamei*	5-HT—female gonadal maturation	Vaca and Alfaro [41]
5	*Procambarus clarkii*	Dopamine—inhibits ovarian maturation 5-HT—stimulates ovarian index and oocyte size; stimulates release of GSH	Sarojini et al. [42]; Luschen et al. [43]
6	*Paratelphusa hydrodromus*	5-HT—stimulates ovarian index in eyestalk ablated animals	Sarojini et al. [39]
7	*Penaeus semisulcatus*	5-HT—stimulates ovarian maturation and spawning	Kumlu [44]
8	*Cherax quadricarinatus*	5-HT—stimulates ovarian maturation in presence of thoracic ganglia	Cahansky et al. [45]
9.	*Scylla serrata*	5-HT—Stimulates reproduction by inducing ecdysteroid and MF secretions.	Girish et al. [46]

Table 1.
The biogenic amines identified and its effect found in different crustacean species. 5-HT: 5-Hydroxytryptamine.

Serotonin induces the release of GSH from thoracic ganglion, whereas dopamine promotes release of eyestalk GIH and reduces thoracic ganglion GSH [47]. The GSH triggered ovarian development by 5-HT in both *in vitro* and *in vivo* is reported in *Penaeus vannamei* [41]. Recently Sainath et al. [38] well demonstrated the reproductive function of serotonin in freshwater rice field crab *O. senex senex*. Since its importance in maturation, biogenic amines are potential candidate molecules for endocrine manipulation of reproduction in crustaceans.

3.2 Gonad stimulating hormone

The gonad stimulating hormone (GSH) is found to be synthesized and released from the crustacean brain and thoracic ganglia. Many *in vivo* and *in vitro* studies have explained the ovarian stimulating effects of brain and thoracic ganglia [48] without isolation and characterization of GSH principle. At first, induced ovarian growth is reported by implanting the brain in *Paratelphusa hydrodromous* [49], later in *Macrobrachium kistnesis, Parapenaeopsis hardwickii* [50, 51]. The stimulatory role of implanted thoracic ganglia is reported for the first time in *Potamon dehaani* [52] and later in *Cherax quadricarinatus* [53]. The combined effect of brain and thoracic ganglia on ovarian development is demonstrated in *P. clarkii* [42]. The role of copper and cadmium on ovarian development through GSH is tested in *Chasmagnathus granulata,* where they incubated ovarian explants and thoracic ganglia along with heavy metals and found inhibition of ovarian maturation [54]. Though the GSH has lots of importance in regulating crustacean reproduction, it could not be used in endocrine manipulation until its structural characterization done in crustaceans.

3.3 Ecdysteroids

In crustaceans, ecdysteroids are polyhydroxylated ketosteoroids synthesized and released from the molting gland called Y-organ with a primary role in regulation of growth. Y-organs are homologous to prothoracic glands of insects and are non-neural paired endocrine glands. Besides molting, ecdysteroids regulate crustacean reproduction and embroyogenesis [55]. The mechanistic action of crustecdysone is explained after the discovery of its receptors called ecdysone receptors (EcR) [56]. EcR binds with retinoid X receptor (RXR) to form heterodimer and stimulates DNA regulatory elements of ecdysteroid signaling pathway [56, 57]. Various physiological functions of ecdysteroids are reported with the EcR and its domain activation, which decides to exert the physiological function by activation or suppression of gene function [58, 59].

At first Charniaux-Cotton and Touir [60] has identified the role of ecdysteroids in the maturation of oocyte of *Lysmata seticaudata* by Y-organectomy, later in *Orchestia gammarella* [32]. The levels of ecdysteroids at the initial stages of spermatogonial mitoses and ovarian maturation are found along with expression of vitellogenin gene in crustaceans [61]. The ecdysteroids and its role is well established in crustaceans. Furthermore, the endocrine manipulation can be executed by supplementing the ecdysteroids through feed to the brood stock to induce reproduction. As a limitation, this method takes longer time to induce ovarian maturation and the animal may enter molt instead of the reproduction.

3.4 Methyl farnesoate

The terpenoid hormone identified through reverse endocrinology is called the methyl farneosate (MF) an analog of insect juvenile hormone III confined only to decapoda and is a secretory product of mandibular organ [62]. MF synthesis and secretion from MO is repressed by eyestalk neuropeptide MOIH [22]. The hemolymph titers of MF are founded high during ovarian maturation and it has a direct relation to promoting maturation in crustaceans [63]. The mechanism of MF induced maturation is found through ecdysteroid synthesis in Y-organs. The mandibular organ disruption due to exposure of environmental pollutants decreases the hemolymph levels of 20-hydroxyecdysone, which is a stimulator product of MF [64]. MF acts as a ligand for retinoid-X-receptor (RXR) and synergize with ecdysteroids to stimulate RXR-EcR heterodimer complex for expression of combined regulatory genes of these two hormones [56, 57]. In *C. maenas* administration of MF elevated the levels of RXR m-RNA in both *in vitro* and *in vivo* [65]. MF is the best suited hormone for endocrine manipulation of reproduction in crustaceans.

4. Conclusion

Seed production is purely done in hatcheries and is supplied to the farmers. Though the reproductive manipulation is not directly influencing the high amount of quality protein production, it is an initial key factor to produce quality feed. The quality seed usage in culture pond is one of the key for high amount of quality protein production. Healthy seed is always superior to maintain and is not easily affected by bacterial, viral and fungal pathogens. More promisingly, superior seed get adjusted easily to new environment and is not affected by fluctuations in the pond management. Moreover, decreased mortality rate in seed, increases the population which reflects the amount of protein/yield at the harvesting time. It is most important that, crustacean hatchery industry should improve the seed quality by following the new methodologies developed

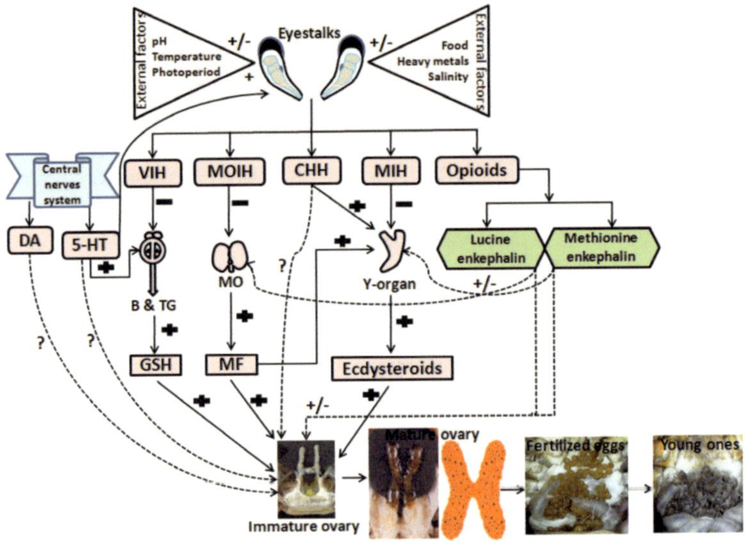

Figure 3.
Influence of internal and external factors in the regulation of crustacean reproduction. DA: Dopamine; 5-HT: 5-Hydroxytryptamine; VIH: Vitellogenesis-inhibiting hormone; MOIH: Mandibular organ-inhibiting hormone; CHH: Crustacean hyperglycemic hormone; MIH: Molt-inhibiting hormone; B & TG: Brain and thoracic ganglia; GSH: Gonad stimulating hormone; MO: Mandibular organ; MF: Methyl farnesoate; '+', '-' and '+/-' denotes activation, inhibition and activation or inhibition, respectively.

from time to time. The systematic pond management and adequate food supply increases protein yield. The high yield influences (increases) the socioeconomic status of farmers ultimately improve the economy of country besides supplementing quality protein forever increasing population. The waste generated (other than protein) in aqua industry is used as feed for poultry, pig, fish and other farm animals, and also in cosmetic industry.

The factors such as pH, temperature, photoperiod, availability of food, salinity of water and heavy metal contamination influences the synthesis and release of CHH-family and other eyestalk secretions in cultured crustaceans.

Regulation of reproduction in crustaceans is a complex process, where a number of internal and external factors are involved. The endocrine hormones and other internal factors act accordingly along with external factors and regulate maturation. The role of well-known internal and external factors is depicted in **Figure 3**. Established endocrine authoritarian mechanisms of crustacean maturation were interpreted in the present chapter. The best method to manipulate endocrine hormones in crustaceans is through supplementation of reproduction positive regulators by means of the feed and is a best alternative for eyestalk ablation technique to improve good quality and quantity of seed from brood stock. Though the administration of positive regulators yielding quality seed, it may injure the animal and increases stress and sometimes it may lead to mortality. The promising method emerging in recent years is gene knockout studies, where the functional genes (negative regulatory genes of reproduction) made inactive. However, knockout studies are not initiated yet in crustacean aquaculture. The identified and reported method for temporary knockdown of gene function in crustaceans is RNAi silencing technology. Silencing of VIH and other genes inhibit reproduction may help to induce maturation thereby quality seed [23]. Controlled external factors with manipulation of internal factors (neither positive nor negative) provide fruitful results without any stress in the brood stock.

Acknowledgements

Author is great full to Prof. P. Sreenivasula Reddy encouragement guidance in successful completion of this Chapter.

Conflict of interest

Authors declare no conflict of interest.

Author details

Ramachandra Reddy Pamuru
Department of Biochemistry, Yogi Vemana University, Kadapa, Andhra Pradesh, India

*Address all correspondence to: reddyprbiotech@gmail.com

References

[1] Panouse JB. Influence de l'ablation du pédoncle oculaire sur la croissance de l'ovaire chez la crevette Leander serratus. Comptes rendus de l'Académie des Sciences. 1943;**217**:553-555

[2] Carlisle DB. Studies on Lysmata seticaudata Risso (Crustacea: Decapoda) V. The ovarian inhibiting hormone and the hormonal inhibition of sex-reversal. Pubblicazioni della Stazione Zoologica di Napoli. 1953;**24**:355-372

[3] Subramoniam T. Mechanisms and control of vitellogenesis in crustaceans. Fisheries Science. 2011;**77**:1-21

[4] Tsukimura B. Crustacean vitellogenesis: Its role in oocyte development. American Zoologist. 2001;**41**:465-476

[5] Reddy PS, Ramamurthi R. Recent trends in crustacean endocrine research. Proceedings of the Indian National Science Academy. 1999;**65**:15-32

[6] Swetha CH, Sainath SB, Reddy PR, Reddy PS. Reproductive endocrinology of female crustaceans: Perspective and prospective. Journal of Marine Science: Research and Development. 2011;**S3**:001

[7] Yang WJ, Aida K, Nagasawa H. Amino acid sequences and activities of multiple hyperglycemic hormones from the kuruma prawn, *Penaeus japonicus*. Peptides. 1997;**18**:479-485

[8] Wilder MN, Okumura T, Tsutsui N. Reproductive mechanisms in crustacea focusing on selected prawn species: Vitellogenin structure, processing and synthetic control. Aqua BioScience Monographs. 2010;**3**:73-110

[9] De Kleijn DP, De Leeuw EP, Van Den Burg BC, Martens GJ, Van Herp F. Cloning and expression of two mRNAs encoding structurally different crustacean hyperglycemic hormone precursors in the lobster *Homarus americanus*. Biochimica et Biophysica Acta. 1995;**1260**:62-66

[10] Soyez D, le Caer JP, Noel PY, Rossier J. Primary structure of two isoforms of the vitellogenesis inhibiting hormone from the lobster *Homarus americanus*. Neuropeptides. 1991;**20**:25-32

[11] Grève P, Sorokine O, Berges T, Lacombe C, Van Dorsselaer A, et al. Isolation and amino acid sequence of a peptide with vitellogenesis inhibiting activity from the terrestrial isopod *Armadillidium vulgare* (Crustacea). General and Comparative Endocrinology. 1999;**115**:406-414

[12] Edomi P, Azzoni E, Mettulio R, Pandolfelli N, Ferrero EA, et al. Gonad inhibiting hormone (GIH) of the Norway lobster (*Nephrops norvegicus*): cDNA cloning, expression, recombinant protein production, and immunolocalization. Gene. 2002;**284**:93-102

[13] Ohira T, Okumura T, Suzuki M, Yajima Y, Tsutsui N, et al. Production and characterization of recombinant vitellogenesis-inhibiting hormone from the American lobster *Homarus americanus*. Peptides. 2006;**27**:1251-1258

[14] Treerattrakool S, Panyim S, Chan SM, Withyachumnarnkul B, Udomkit A. Molecular characterization of gonad-inhibiting hormone of *Penaeus monodon* and elucidation of its inhibitory role in vitellogenin expression by RNA interference. FEBS Journal. 2008;**275**:970-980

[15] Okumura T. Effects of cyclic nucleotides, calcium ionophore, and phorbol ester on vitellogenin mRNA levels in incubated ovarian fragments of the kuruma prawn *Marsupenaeus japonicus*. General and Comparative Endocrinology. 2006;**148**:245-251

[16] Okumura T. Intracellular signaling pathways for vitellogenin synthesis in the ovary of the kuruma prawn, *Penaeus (marsupenaeus) japonicus*. Bulletin of Fisheries Research Agency. 2008;**26**:135-141. (in Japanese)

[17] Wainwright G, Webster SG, Wilkinson MC, Chung JS, Rees HH. Structure and significance of mandibular organ-inhibiting hormone in the crab, Cancer pagurus. Involvement in multihormonal regulation of growth and reproduction. The Journal of Biological Chemistry. 1996;**271**:12749-12754

[18] Tsukimura B, Borst DW. Regulation of methyl farnesoate in the hemolymph and mandibular organ of the lobster, *Homarus americanus*. General and Comparative Endocrinology. 1992;**2**:296-303

[19] Chaves AR. Effects of sinus gland extract on mandibular organ size and methyl farnesoate synthesis in the crayfish. Comparative Biochemistry and Physiology. Part A: Molecular and Integrative Physiology. 2001;**128**:327-333

[20] Waddy SL, Aiken DE, De Kleijn DPV. Control of reproduction. In: Factor JR, editor. Biology of the lobster, *Homarus americanus*. San Diego, USA: Academic Press; 1995. pp. 217-266

[21] Borst DW, Tsukimura B, Laufer H, Couch E. Regional differences in methyl farnesoate production by the lobster mandibular organ. The Biological Bulletin. 1994;**186**:916

[22] Nagaraju GPC, Reddy PR, Reddy PS. Mandibular organ: It's relation to body weight, sex, molt and reproduction in the crab, Oziotelphusa senex senex Fabricius (1791). Aquaculture. 2004;**232**:603-612

[23] Lugo JM, Morera Y, Rodríguez T, Huberman A, Ramos L, et al. Molecular cloning and characterization of the crustacean hyperglycemic hormone cDNA from *Litopenaeus schmitti*; functional analysis by double stranded RNA interference technique. FEBS Journal. 2006;**273**:5669-5677

[24] De Kleijn DP, Janssen KP, Waddy SL, Hegeman R, Lie WY, et al. Expression of the crustacean hyperglycemic hormones and the gonad inhibiting hormone during the reproductive cycle of the female American lobster *Homarus americanus*. Journal of Endocrinology. 1998;**156**:291-298

[25] Gu PL, Yu KL, Chan SM. Molecular characterization of an additional shrimp hyperglycemic hormone: cDNA cloning, gene organization, expression and biological assay of recombinant proteins. FEBS Letters. 2000;**472**:122-128

[26] Van Herp F. Molecular, cytological and physiological aspects of the crustacean hyperglycemic hormone family. In: Cost EM, Webster SG, editors. Recent Advances in Arthropod Endocrinology. Vol. 65. Cambridge, UK: University Press; 1998. pp. 53-70

[27] Chung JS, Webster SG. Moult cycle-related changes in biological activity of moult-inhibiting hormone (MIH) and crustacean hyperglycaemic hormone (CHH) in the crab, *Carcinus maenas*. From target to transcript. European Journal of Biochemistry. 2003;**270**:3280-3288

[28] Zarubin TP, Chang ES, Mykles DL. Expression of recombinant eyestalk crustacean hyperglycemic hormone from the tropical land crab, *Gecarcinus lateralis*, that inhibits Y-organ ecdysteroidogenesis in vitro. Molecular Biology Reports. 2009;**36**:1231-1237

[29] Tiu SH, Chan SM. The use of recombinant protein and RNA interference approaches to study the reproductive functions of a

gonad-stimulating hormone from the shrimp *Metapenaeus ensis*. FEBS Journal. 2007;**274**:4385-4395

[30] Zmora N, Trant J, Zohar Y, Chung JS. Molt-inhibiting hormone stimulates vitellogenesis at advanced ovarian developmental stages in the female blue crab, Callinectes sapidus 1: An ovarian stage dependent involvement. Saline Systems. 2009;**5**:7

[31] Gu PL, Tobe SS, Chow BKC, Chu KH, He JG, Chan S-M. Characterization of an additional molt inhibiting hormonelike neuropeptide from the shrimp *Metapenaeus ensis*. Peptides. 2002;**23**:1875-1883

[32] Meusy JJ, Blanche MF, Junera H. Molting and vitellogenesis in the crustacean amphipod Orchestia gammarella Pallas. II. Synthesis of vitellogenin (female protein fraction of hemolymph) after the destruction of Y organs. General and Comparative Endocrinology. 1977;**33**:35-40

[33] Kishori B, Reddy PS. Antagonistic effects of opioid peptides in the regulation of ovarian growth of the Indian rice field crab, Oziotelphusa senex senex Fabricius. Invertebrate Reproduction and Development. 2000;**37**:107-111

[34] Kishori B, Reddy PS. Influence of leucine-enkephalin on moulting and vitellogenesis in the freshwater crab, Oziotelphusa senex senex (Fabricius, 1791) (Decapoda, Brachyura). Crustaceana. 2004;**76**:1281-1290

[35] Reddy PS. Involvement of opioid peptides in the regulation of reproduction in the prawn *Penaeus indicus*. Naturwissenschaften. 2000;**87**:535-538

[36] Keller R, Beyer J. Zur hyperglyka¨mischen Wirkung von Serotonin und Augenstiel extrakt beimFlußkrebs *Orconectes limosus*. Zeitschrift für vergleichende Physiologie. 1968;**59**:78-85

[37] Richardson HG, Deecaraman M, Fingerman M. The effect of biogenic amines on ovarian development in fiddler crab, Uca pugilator. Comparative Biochemistry and Physiology. 1991;**99**:53-56

[38] Sainath SB, Reddy PS. Effect of selected biogenic amines on reproduction in the freshwater edible crab Oziotelphusa senex senex. Aquaculture. 2011;**313**:144-148

[39] Sarojini R, Nagabhushanam R, Fingerman M. Evidence for opioid involvement in the regulation ofovarian maturation of the fiddler crab, Uca pugilator. Comparative Biochemistry and Physiology. 1995a;**111A**:279-282

[40] Makkapan W, Maikaeo L, Miyazaki T, Chotigeat W. Molecular mechanism of serotonin via methyl farnesoate in ovarian development of white shrimp: Fenneropenaeus merguiensis de Man. Aquaculture. 2011;**321**:101-107

[41] Vaca A, Alfaro AJ. Ovarian maturation and spawning in the white shrimp, Penaeus vannamei, by serotonin injection. Aquaculture. 2000;**182**:373-385

[42] Sarojini R, Nagabhushanam R, Fingerman M. Mode of action of the neurotransmitter 5-hydroxytryptamine in stimulating ovarian maturation in the red swamp crayfish, *Procambarus clarkii*: An in vivo and in vitro study. Journal of Experimental Zoology. 1995b;**271**:395-400

[43] Luschen W, Wilig A, Jaros PP. The role of biogenic amines in the control of blood glucose level in the decapod crustacean *Carcinus maenas L*. Comparative Biochemistry and Physiology. 1993;**105**:291-296

[44] Kumlu M. Gonadal maturation and spawning in Penaeus semisulcatus de Hann, 1844 by hormone injection. Turkish Journal of Zoology. 2005;**29**:193-199

[45] Cahansky AV, Medesani DA, Chaulet A, Rodríguez EM. In vitro effects of both dopaminergic and enkephalinergic antagonists on the ovarian growth of *Cherax quadricarinatus* (Decapoda, Parastacidae), at different periods of the reproductive cycle. Comparative Biochemistry and Physiology Part A: Molecular and Integrative Physiology. 2011;**158**:126-131

[46] Girish BP, Swetha CH, Reddy PS. Serotonin induces ecdysteroidogenesis and methyl farnesoate synthesis in the mud crab, *Scylla serrata*. Biochemical and Biophysical Research Communication. 2017;**490**:1340-1345

[47] Fingerman M. Roles of neurotransmitters in regulating reproductive hormone release and gonadal maturation in decapod crustaceans. Invertebrate Reproduction and Development. 1997;**31**:47-54

[48] Chang ES. Hormonal control of molting in decapod crustacea. American Zoologist. 1985;**25**:179-185

[49] Gomez R. Acceleration of development of gonads by implantations of brain in the crab *Paratelphusa hydrodromous*. Naturwiss. 1965;**52**:216

[50] Sarojini R, Mirajkar MS, Nagabhushanam R. Bihormonal control of oogenesis in the freshwater prawn, *Macrobrachium kistnensis*. Acta Physiologica Hungarica. 1983;**61**:5-10

[51] Kulkarni G, Nagabhushanam R, Joshi P. Effect of progesterone on ovarian maturation in a marine penaeid prawn *Parapenaeopsis hardwickii* (Miers, 1878). Indian Journal of Experimental Biology. 1979;**17**:986-987

[52] Otsu T. Bihormonal control of sexual cycle in the freshwater crab, *Potoman dehaani*. Embryologia. 1963;**8**:1-20

[53] Von Hentig R. Influence of salinity and temperature on development, growth, reproduction and energy budget of Artemia Salina. Marine Biology. 1971;**9**:145-182

[54] Medesani DA, López Greco LS, Rodríguez EM. Interference of cadmium and copper with the endocrine control of ovarian growth, in the estuarine crab *Chasmagnathus granulata*. Aquatic Toxicology. 2004;**69**:165-174

[55] Subramoniam T. Crustacean ecdysteroids in reproduction and embryogenesis. Comparative Biochemistry and Physiology. 2000;**125**:135-156

[56] Tarrant AM, Behrendt L, Stegeman JJ, Verslycke T. Ecdysteroid receptor from the American lobster *Homarus americanus*: EcR/RXR isoform cloning and ligand-binding properties. General and Comparative Endocrinology. 2011;**173**:346-355

[57] Hill RJ, Billas IM, Bonneton F, Graham LD, Lawrence MC. Ecdysone receptors: From the Ashburner model to structural biology. Annual Review of Entomology. 2013;**58**:251-271

[58] Tan A, Palli SR. Ecdysone receptor isoforms play distinct roles in controlling molting and metamorphosis in the red floor beatle, *Tribolium castaneum*. Molecular and Cellular Endocrinology. 2008;**291**:42-49

[59] Schwedes C, Tulsiani S, Carney GE. Ecdysone receptor expression and activity in adult *Drosophila melanogaster*. Journal of Insect Physiology. 2011;**57**:899-907

[60] Charniaux-Cotton H, Toui A. Contrale de la prgvitellogenese et

de la vitellogenese chez la crevette hermaphrodite Lysmata seticaudata Risso. Comptes rendus de l'Académie des Sciences. 1973;**276**:2717-2720

[61] Tiu SH, Chan SM, Tobe SS. The effects of farnesoic acid and 20-hydroxyecdysone on vitellogenin gene expression in the lobster, *Homarus americanus*, and possible roles in the reproductive process. General and Comparative Endocrinology. 2010;**166**:337-345

[62] Laufer H, Biggers WJ, Ahl JS. Stimulation of ovarian maturation in the crayfish *Procambarus clarkii* by methyl farnesoate. General and Comparative Endocrinology. 1998;**111**:113-118

[63] Reddy PR, Nagaraju GPC, Reddy PS. Involvement of methyl farnesoate in the regulation of molting and reproduction in the freshwater crab Oziotelphusa senex senex. Journal of Crustacean Biology. 2004;**24**:511-515

[64] Hyne RV. Review of the reproductive biology of amphipods and their endocrine regulation: Identification of mechanistic pathways for reproductive toxicants. Environmental Toxicology and Chemistry. 2011;**30**:2647-2657

[65] Nagaraju GPC. Reproductive regulators in decapod crustaceans: An overview. Journal of Experimental Biology. 2011;**214**:3-16